Contents

Sexual

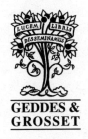

FAMILY · MEDICAL

Health

GEDDES &
GROSSET

Published 2002 by Geddes & Grosset
David Dale House, New Lanark ML11 9DJ, Scotland
© Geddes & Grosset 2002

The material contained in this book is set out in good faith for
general guidance only. Whilst every effort has been made to ensure
that the information in this book is accurate, relevant and up to date,
this book is sold on the condition that neither the author nor the
publisher can be found legally responsible for the consequences
of any errors or omissions.

ISBN 1 84205 104 0
Printed and bound in the UK

NB: Words in SMALL CAPS within the main text indicate important terms or topics that are commonly dealt with in more detail within a relevant section of the book.

CHAPTER 1

Introduction

In Western countries, people are bombarded with explicit information and images about sex to such an extent that it is difficult to avoid exposure to such material. In view of this, it might be expected that from a relatively young age everyone would be well informed about matters concerning their sexual and reproductive health.

However, surveys reveal a somewhat different story, which is that on a personal level, people may be quite ill informed about this important aspect of their own health. Unfortunately, ignorance or carelessness with regard to sexual heath all too often results in considerable physical and emotional suffering with unwanted pregnancies, damaging and potentially life-threatening infections and diseases, and infertility being just some of the consequences of being ill informed.

The ramifications of sexual and reproductive health extend, in a sometimes surprising way, into all the corners of human experience. The purpose of this book is to review and present in a straightforward manner, the information that we all need to know to safeguard not only our own health, but that of our family and those who are closest to us. The saying that 'to be forewarned is to be forearmed' could have been invented with sexual and reproductive health in mind. It is hoped that by reading this book, your own knowledge and understanding will be enriched, helping you to feel better equipped to protect your health.

HUMAN SEXUAL BEHAVIOUR – OURSELVES AND OTHER ANIMALS

Among the number of distinctive features which set the human species apart from nearly all other animals is our sexuality and reproductive behaviour. Almost all other animals (with a few exceptions, particularly among our closest relatives, the primates) mate for the sole purpose of producing young. Most of these animals confine mating to a brief breeding season and others may only be sexually receptive for one or two days in the year. Hence in these animals, sexual behaviour simply does not take place outside these clearly defined periods of time.

In contrast, human beings can 'mate' at any time, the only limiting factors being individual psychological and physical preferences and the operation of social constraints. In addition, human beings possess a unique cycle of sexual response which is activated by a variety of pleasurable stimuli involving most of the senses. In the achievement of orgasm, which is the climax of the sexual response cycle in both men and women, human beings apparently gain greater pleasure in the sexual act than almost all other animals.

In most animals, mating results in the production of offspring, the nurturing of which is a physically demanding and energy-exhausting exercise requiring fitness and the availability of a good supply of food. This means that for animals, it makes sense to limit the sexual act to a particular period or breeding cycle, usually seasonally timed so that young will be born when food is plentiful, thus giving parents and offspring the greatest chance of survival.

At some point in human evolution, a highly attuned and pleasurable sexual response behaviour developed, presumably to enhance reproductive success. Its existence means that human beings readily engaged in sexual activity, not only for procreation but also for pleasure – something which is too great a risk for most other animals. For early human beings, the sexual act would have resulted in the expectation, if not the actual result, of pregnancy and the birth of a child.

However, historical evidence suggests that different peoples have always, to a great or lesser extent, attempted to divorce sex from procreation by employing means to control their own fertility. Of course, it has only been with the development of effective means of contraception that this has become reliably feasible. Hence, the people of today who have easy access to information and contraception are able to engage in sex without the consequent risk of pregnancy. There is no doubt that this has brought about a revolution in attitudes, both amongst individuals and within society as a whole, making it possible for people to engage in sex whenever they wish, without even considering its natural consequences.

However, in spite of this detachment in our thinking, in humans as in other animals, sex evolved for the purpose of procreation. The following chapters, describing the anatomy and function of the reproductive system (in which humans share more similarities than differences when compared to other mammals) is therefore fundamental for any book examining sexual and reproductive health.

CHAPTER 2

The male
reproductive system

The male and female reproductive systems consist of the organs, glands and supporting structures which produce, release and transport reproductive cells (gametes) along with the hormones which control the process and are responsible for sexual maturation at **PUBERTY**. Coitus, copulation or sexual intercourse between male and female makes it possible for the gametes (the female egg and male sperm) to meet, fuse and create a new life in the form of an embryo. This embryo contains a unique combination of genes which are derived equally from both parents, enabling genetic information to be passed from one generation to another.

THE ANATOMY OF THE MALE
REPRODUCTIVE SYSTEM

The male reproductive system comprises internal organs including a pair of testes (*sing.* testis) or testicles, together with accessory ducts and sex glands and

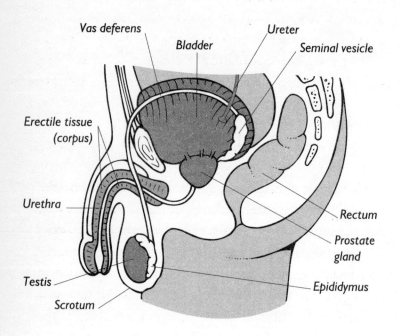

The male reproductive system

supporting structures or external genitalia – the scrotum and penis.

The paired testicles lie within the scrotum which is a pouch or sac of wrinkled, loose skin situated outside the main part of the body. The scrotum is divided internally into two cavities or sacs by a septum – a thin, planar 'wall' or partition of tissue. Each sac contains a testicle which is an oval-shaped gland of approximately 5 cm in length. During foetal development, the testicles are formed in the abdominal wall and descend to their final position during the seventh month of pregnancy via paired passages called the inguinal canals which open into the scrotum on either side. Occasionally, one testicle may fail to descend normally – a condition known as CRYPTORCHIDISM.

The temperature inside the scrotum is about 2° C lower than that of the abdomen, since it is situated externally. This is vital for the production and storage of sperm – processes which are inhibited at normal body temperature. Each testicle has an outer, membranous double layer called the tunica vaginalis which surrounds an inner, fibrous membrane, the tunica albuginea, which protects the gland. The bulk of the testicle consists of numerous, fine convoluted tubules, the seminiferous tubules, which, if collectively extended and joined, would be about 500 metres in length.

The seminiferous tubules are supported by connective tissue and lined with cells that produce the sex cells, the spermatozoa. The connective tissue contains nerves and blood vessels which supply the testicle and also cells of Leydig which are responsible for the production of hormones. The cells are interspersed with larger sertoli cells that provide support and nourishment for immature spermatozoa (spermatids). The seminiferous tubules are divided into compartments which unite to form larger ducts and tubules, eventually connecting with the epididymis.

This is a larger, highly folded tube which, if extended, would be about 7 metres in length and it acts as a reservoir in which sperm mature and are stored. The epididymis is lined with smooth muscle, the contractions of which propel mature sperm during ejaculation towards and into a long, muscular tube called the vas deferens. The paired vasa deferentia ascend from each testicle on either side into the abdomen and around and behind the bladder, before beginning to descend once again. They are important accessory organs of the male reproductive system, each measuring approximately 45 cm in length, which effectively join the testicles with the urethra. They convey sperm by muscular movements (peristalsis) towards the urethra.

A pair of important glands, the seminal vesicles, are situated below and behind the bladder and each empties, via a series of ducts, into the lower part of the vas deferens on either side. The ducts from these glands along with the final portion of the vas deferens, unite to form a short ejaculatory duct – a tube which opens into the urethra at its lower end. The ejaculatory ducts from either side open into the urethra at about the same level. Above this junction, the highest portion of the urethra leads into the urinary bladder.

The seminal vesicles secrete important substances to nourish and support the sperm. Their secretions account for about 60 per cent of the constituents of semen – the fluid which passes out of the penis during ejaculation. Seminal gland secretions are clear and viscous and contain fructose (fruit sugar) which provides additional energy for the sperm, amino acids (proteins), prostaglandins (hormone-like substances) and mucus. Prostaglandins have a local effect on the muscles of the female womb, causing them to contract and hence aid the upward passage of sperm. Amino acids cause coagulation of the fluid semen, so that the muscular contractions of the uterus are rendered more effective.

The urethra is a tube or duct which serves both the urinary system and the reproductive system in the human male (but not in the female). Its total length is about 20 cm and, because it passes through three distinct regions, it can be subdivided into the prostatic urethra, membranous urethra and penile urethra. The prostatic urethra is the uppermost portion which is surrounded by the prostate gland. This is the largest of the male accessory sexual glands and is roughly spherical, about the size of a walnut. It is located immediately below the bladder, surrounding the neck of that organ and also the ejaculatory ducts. It opens via several small ducts directly into the urethra and secretes an alkaline, milky fluid which is added as a constituent to the semen. The effect of the prostatic secretion is to create an environment favourable to the survival of sperm by counteracting the natural acidity present in the vagina.

Beyond the prostate gland, the membranous urethra forms a relatively short section of the duct before continuing through the penis as the penile urethra which is about 15 to 20 cm in length. This exits to the outside through the external urethral orifice (opening) at the base of the penis. Below the prostate gland and situated slightly above the base of the penis, lie a third pair of small, accessory sexual glands, the bulbo-urethral or Cowper's glands. These peanut-sized glands release a small quantity of sticky, clear secretion containing a few sperm into the urethra, each via a single duct, just before ejaculation. It has been suggested that this fluid acts as a lubricant for the end of the penis and/or has a protective function for sperm but its significance is unclear. However, the fact that a secretion containing sperm is emitted before ejaculation means that the withdrawal method of CONTRACEPTION cannot be relied upon.

The release of all the various constituents of semen is known as emission and it normally precedes ejaculation and orgasm which depend primarily upon responses in the penis. The penis is largely composed of three cylindrical layers of spongy, erectile tissue called cavernous bodies which are themselves modified blood vessels (capillaries and veins). The innermost layer is a cylindrical blood sinus or chamber called the corpus spongiosum which encloses the urethra. At the base of the penis near to the body it expands to form the urethral bulb and at the lower end or head, it widens to become the glans penis. The glans is covered by a layer of thin skin which is highly sensitive and which is folded to form a retractable layer called the prepuce or foreskin. Two further cylinders or blood sinuses called the corpora cavernosa (*sing.* corpus cavernosum) make up the rest of the erectile tissue of the penis.

Usually, the corpora are flat and so the penis is limp and flaccid. During sexual arousal, which occurs as a result of tactile and visual stimulation, a rush of blood floods into the cavernosa producing engorgement and a consequent expansion in size and rigidity, namely an erection. Contraction of muscles at the base of the penis prevent the blood from escaping so aiding the continuation of the erection. Further stimulation, brought about by the rhythmic movements of the penis during sexual intercourse, normally result in ejaculation and orgasm.

Ejaculation is the term commonly used to describe the sudden pumping out of semen from the urethral orifice of the penis. The semen released at each ejaculation contains about 400 million mature sperm cells, hence **SPERMATOGENESIS** (the production of sperm) occurs continuously in the adult male. Orgasm describes the same event but is popularly used in reference to the pleasurable feelings and sensations of sexual climax in both males and females. In males, ejaculation/orgasm is a reflex activity caused by the contraction of muscles not only in the penis but also in the lower abdomen, pelvis and buttocks. Part of this reflex also involves the contraction of the sphincter muscle at the base of the bladder, which prevents urine from passing into the urethra during the event.

Following orgasm, the penis rapidly decreases in size as muscles relax and blood drains out of the corpora. A refractory period follows during which further stimulation will not produce an erection. This is a natural, physiological state of nerve and muscle cells following the passage of electrical impulses and contraction. It is the period of recovery when the chemical balance is being restored to cell membranes and it is impossible for a nerve or muscle cell to respond to further stimulus. In young men, the overall refractory period is usually short-lived but it may lengthen with increasing age.

HORMONAL CONTROL AND SPERMATOGENESIS
HORMONAL CONTROL
The most important sex hormones in the male are collectively known as androgens and out of these, the one that plays the largest part is testosterone. Androgens are mainly secreted by the interstitial cells of Leydig in the testicles and are steroid hormones that

have potent effects within the body. They are responsible for the development of the primary and secondary sexual characteristics at **PUBERTY**, i.e. the maturation of the sexual organs and the appearance of adult male features. In addition, androgens have a role in sperm production in the determination of sex drive or libido and in the occurrence of other behaviours such as aggressiveness. Androgens are additionally released in much smaller amounts by other endocrine (hormone-secreting) structures, namely the cortex of the paired adrenal glands located on the upper surface of each kidney.

The release of androgens from the testicles is mediated by structures which are located far away at the base of the brain – the hypothalamus and the pituitary gland. The hypothalamus is an area of the brain lying beneath the cerebrum and thalamus which has a wide variety of regulatory functions. Included in these is the production and release of two sets of hormones which are transported to the pituitary gland, located at the base of the hypothalamus. The most important group as far as the male reproductive system is concerned are called releasing factors or gonadotrophin releasing hormone (GNRH) which act on the anterior (frontal) part of the pituitary gland.

The pituitary gland or hypophysis is a small but vitally important endocrine gland which has two lobes, the anterior adenohypophysis and the posterior neurohypophysis. The neurohypophysis stores and one of which, vasopressin or antidiuretic hormone, reduces urine secretion by increasing the quantity of water reabsorbed from the blood by the kidneys. The adenohypophysis is prompted to produce and release a number of different hormones under the influence of releasing factors received from the hypothalamus, including the gonadotrophins or gonadotrophic hormones which act directly on the testicles.

Luteinizing hormone (LH) or interstitial cell stimulating hormone (ICSH), as it may be designated in males, acts on the cells of Leydig and causes them to produce androgens. Follicle stimulating hormone (FSH) acts on the cells of the seminiferous tubules, causing them to produce sperm by the process known as **SPERMATOGENESIS** (*see* below). The level of circulating androgens in the blood regulates the release of GNRH, ICSH and FSH and this information is interpreted in the brain. GNRH release is additionally regulated by the level of ICSH and FSH. These controlling mechanisms are highly complex and have the effect of keeping hormone levels fairly constant in human males.

This is not the case in many other male mammals where hormone release is associated with breeding cycles (*see* **HUMAN SEXUAL BEHAVIOUR — OURSELVES AND OTHER MAMMALS**). Through their operation, it can be seen that ICSH has an indirect effect on spermatogenesis through androgen production while FSH controls it directly. Occasionally, hormonal imbalance or deficiencies arising, for example, as a result of disorders in the pituitary gland, can be a cause of IMPOTENCE or INFERTILITY in men when there is nothing wrong with the reproductive organs themselves.

SPERMATOGENESIS

Spermatogenesis describes the means by which mature spermatozoa (sperm) are produced in the testicles, a process which begins at puberty and continues throughout life. Primary germ cells are present in the testicles of a male foetus and these develop into immature, precursor sperm called spermatogonia. Spermatogonia are present near the outer wall of the seminiferous tubules and they undergo many divisions by a process known as mitosis to produce a large reservoir of potential sperm. Spermatogonia contain the full (diploid) number of chromosomes which are identical to those contained in every cell of that individual. At puberty, a proportion of these cells become active and undergo further differentiation and mitotic (by mitosis) division to become primary spermatocytes which are still diploid. In an adult man, about 3 million spermatozoa undergo this process every day.

During the next stage, the primary spermatocytes undergo a specialized process of division which takes place in two stages, and is called meiosis. The first

Spermatogenesis and spermiogenesis in relation to the structure of a seminiferous tubule.

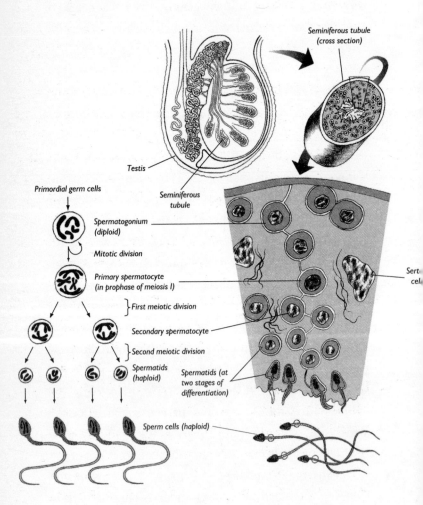

meiotic division produces cells called secondary spermatocytes and the second one cells named spermatids which are immature sperm. The critical factor about meiosis is that once the divisions have been completed, the spermatids are haploid, i.e. they possess half the number of chromosomes (which carry the genes) of the original spermatogonia. Exactly the same process occurs in OOGENESIS in the female, ensuring that human eggs or ova are also haploid. By this means, when sperm and egg unite at FERTILIZATION, the newly created potential human being has its own unique, diploid combination of chromosomes, half derived from the father and half from the mother, which determines all the characteristics of the individual.

The haploid spermatids next undergo a process of differentiation and maturation called spermiogenesis during which they associate with, and are nourished by, the sertoli cells of the seminiferous tubules. During the whole process of spermatogenesis, the developing cells are gradually moved downwards towards the lumen or central space of the seminiferous tubules. Eventually, they enter the lumen and migrate to the epididymis where, now as mature sperm, they acquire the ability to move. The whole developmental process takes about 70 days in a human male.

The spermatozoon or sperm is the mature reproductive cell or gamete and it can be visualized as being somewhat like a tadpole with a head, mid-piece and

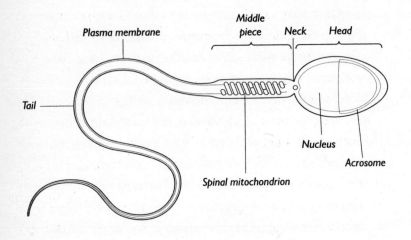

The structure of a human spermatozoon

tail. The head encloses the haploid nucleus containing half the number of chromosomes, tipped at the front by a thickened structure called the acrosome. This contains enzymes which help the sperm to penetrate an egg. Behind the head lies the mid-piece or middle section containing a large, coiled energy-producing organelle called a mitochondrion. This provides the necessary energy for the movement of the spermatozoon once it has been released into the female vagina. Most mammalian sperm contain many mitochondria but in humans and some other species there is a single, large mitochondrion.

Behind the mid-piece there is a long, thin tail consisting of a plasma membrane surrounding a flagellum, a thread-like structure which lashes from side to side to produce forward movement. Individual sperm are minute, measuring about 4 micrometres and several million would fit onto the head of a pin. Once ejaculated into the vagina, each sperm, along with millions of others, swims and is moved upwards, at a rate of 1.5 to 3 mm per minute, high into the female reproductive tract. Sperm retain their ability to move for several days but quickly lose their ability to penetrate an egg. Hence only the 'fittest' sperm are able to attempt **FERTILIZATION**.

CHAPTER 3

Diseases and disorders of the male reproductive system and their treatment

The male reproductive organs and genitalia are subject to various diseases and disorders, some of which are more common than others. A familiarity with and understanding of these conditions should be essential knowledge for every young man (and those concerned about him) from the time of puberty, so that he is better able to protect his health.

Infections which affect the reproductive organs can be roughly grouped into two categories, although there is some overlap between them. The first group are those which are most commonly acquired as a result of sexual activity and include the classic **SEXUALLY TRANSMITTED DISEASES** or **STDS**. These are fully described in Chapter 11.

The second group include infections which are not necessarily acquired by sexual intimacy but may be contracted by other means. This group, along with congenital (inborn) structural and cancerous disorders of the reproductive organs, are described in the following sections. They are grouped according to the organs which they affect.

TESTICLES

CRYPTORCHIDISM OR UNDESCENDED TESTICLE

Cryptorchidism describes the condition in which one (or rarely both) testicle has failed to descend from the abdomen into the scrotum of a newborn baby boy. In most cases, the testicle descends spontaneously in the infant's first year of life and may even descend and retract one or more times. However, if it has not permanently descended by the child's first birthday, corrective surgery is needed which is normally performed before the age of three years. The operation performed is called orchidopexy or testicle fixation and it is performed under general anaesthetic. A small incision is made in the scrotum and the testicle, along with its associated blood vessels and nerves, is carefully brought down into its correct position and secured by means of stitches so that there is no possibility of retraction. The external wound is then stitched and the child normally recovers quickly and completely within a short space of time.

The cause of cryptorchidism is unknown but is believed to be related to hormonal influences during foetal development. The condition appears to be becoming more prevalent and there is concern that this is connected with maternal exposure to environmental chemicals, some of which mimic hormone activity. However, there is little available advice for expectant mothers on how they might be able to limit risks.

It is essential that an undescended testicle is treated early and well before **PUBERTY**, because it cannot function at the prevailing body temperature within the abdomen. It is felt that the optimum time is between the age of two and three when the child is less likely to feel embarrassment or suffer psychological trauma and will forget about the operation as he grows older. An undescended testicle, even when treated early, increases the risk of testicular cancer hence it is essential for an affected individual to be vigilant in carrying out **TESTICULAR SELF-EXAMINATION**.

ORCHITIS (INFLAMMATION OF THE TESTICLES)

Orchitis (inflammation of the testicles) is an intensely painful condition in which there is redness, heat and swelling of the testicles and scrotum. There is usually an initial build-up of symptoms and it is essential to seek immediate medical treatment if pain or discomfort is noticed in this region. As with so many other conditions, the earlier treatment begins the sooner the condition can be cured. Orchitis is most commonly associated with **GONORRHOEA** (*see* Chapter 11) but there are other causes as well. They include inflammation and infections of the bladder and urinary organs such as bladder stones and cystitis, mumps and tuberculosis. Treatment involves bed rest, the use of support bandages and possibly ice packs to reduce inflammation, strong pain-relieving drugs and, if infection is involved, courses of antibiotics. In severe cases, admittance to hospital may be necessary where morphine may be administered to relieve pain.

TESTICULAR TORSION

Testicular torsion occurs as a result of a twisting of the spermatic cord (**VAS DEFERENS**, nerves and blood vessels) which supplies each testicle, threatening damage to the affected testicle and causing intense pain. Testicular torsion usually occurs on one side only and generally the cause is unclear although it may result from injury such as that which may be sustained from playing vigorous sports. There is sudden, often severe pain followed by a possible rise in temperature, sweating, accelerated heartbeat, nausea and vomiting. This is an emergency condition which requires immediate admittance to hospital for assessment and treatment. Except in the mildest cases, treatment is likely to involve surgery to untangle the spermatic cord and to attach the testicle to the wall of the scrotum to prevent a recurrence. If treatment is delayed, the testicle may be irreparably damaged due to the interruption in its blood and nerve supply. If this occurs, orchidectomy – surgical removal of the testicle and spermatic cord – becomes necessary. Although unpleasant, this surgery does not affect sexual function and enjoyment or fertility.

SPERMATOCOELE

A spermatocoele is a benign, cyst-like lump in the scrotal sac, which is derived from the EPIDIDYMIS and contains sperm and can be felt externally. Usually some fluid is aspirated from the cyst to confirm the diagnosis and it is then surgically removed, this being a relatively minor procedure.

TESTICULAR CANCER (CANCER OF THE TESTICLE)

There are several forms of malignant tumour which can affect the testicles, two of the most important of which are seminoma and teratoma. A seminoma is believed to be derived from the epithelium of the SEMINIFEROUS TUBULES. A teratoma is a tumour that is composed of unusual tissues not normally found at that site and derived from partially developed embryological cells. A teratoma can develop in a testicle and particularly in one that was undescended (*see* CRYPTORCHIDISM). In recent years, there has been an increase in the number of male infants born with an undescended testicle and this condition, even when corrected by early surgery, produces a five-fold increase in the risk of cancer.

Testicular cancer can occur in any male past **PUBERTY** but teratoma is most common in young men between the ages of 20 and 35 and is not unheard of in teenage boys. There is evidence that there are genetic factors involved in some cases of testicular cancer with risks increasing if a close male relative (father or brother) has been affected. Most forms of the disease respond well to treatment if detected at an early stage but a few are highly malignant. Symptoms can be few and go unnoticed but when they do occur include a dull ache in the scrotum or a feeling of heaviness and/or a detectable lump or a change in the external appearance of the testicles within the scrotal sac. Most irregularities or lumps are benign but anyone who notices anything unusual should seek medical advice without delay. In the event of testicular cancer being diagnosed, often by means of a biopsy (the examination, usually under a microscope, of a sample of tissue from a lump) and blood tests, surgery and possibly chemotherapy and/or radiotherapy are likely to be employed. If detected early, surgery alone is often sufficient and this could consist of the removal of the lump (lumpectomy) or the complete removal of the affected testicle (orchidectomy). Recovery after surgery is usually swift and without complications and all that is required thereafter is a periodic check-up to ensure that the cancer has not returned or spread. Removal of one testicle does not affect sexual function or enjoyment or the ability to father children.

Regular **TESTICULAR SELF-EXAMINATION** should become a matter of routine for all males from the age of 15 years upwards.

VARICOCOELE

A varicocoele is a group of distended veins in the spermatic cord causing a soft swelling and occasionally discomfort or aching. In some cases, it may also cause a poor sperm count and affect fertility and this may necessitate surgical removal of the varicocoele (varicocoelectomy).

PROSTATE GLAND

BENIGN PROSTATIC HYPERTROPHY (BPH)

Benign prostatic hypertrophy (BPH) is the medical name for the enlargement of the prostate gland that is a common condition among middle-aged and elderly men. The condition causes pressure to be exerted on the neck of the bladder which obstructs the normal flow of urine. The bladder consequently extends and there is a frequent need to urinate, especially at night, with discomfort or pain and only a weak flow or 'dribbling'. Since the bladder is not being emptied efficiently, infections may occur and rarely this may involve the upper urinary tract and kidneys.

Symptoms associated with this condition should always be investigated and the patient is usually referred to a urology clinic where physical examination, along with blood and urine tests, will establish the diagnosis. Thorough investigation is needed in order to rule out any possibility of malignancy.

The condition is normally a progressive one but drug treatments may help for a time as may limiting the consumption of drinks in the evening. Eventually, surgical removal of the prostate gland or prostatectomy becomes necessary. The surgery is commonly performed via the urethra using a fine instrument which destroys the gland, the particles then being flushed to the outside. This means that there is no wound and recovery after the operation is normally rapid following a short stay in hospital.

Excess alcohol consumption and many prescription drugs increase the risk of BPH, but this is an extremely common condition of older age. Maintaining physical fitness, having an active sex life and limiting the drinking of alcohol may reduce the risk of this troublesome condition arising.

PROSTATITIS

Prostatitis refers to inflammation, usually accompanied by, and caused by, bacterial infection which may gain access from the exterior via the urethra. Symptoms include frequency of urination accompanied by a burning sensation and pain, inability to empty the bladder completely and difficulty in starting to urinate. Also, there may be generalized aches and pains, but especially in the lower back and pelvis, fever, chills and occasionally, blood in the urine. The risk of contracting the condition increases if there has been a recent infection of the urinary tract or if the man is a smoker and/or heavy drinker. An active sex life is believed to decrease the risk. Treatment involves bed rest and courses of antibiotics along with pain-relieving drugs. If the infection is very severe, admittance to hospital may be necessary and there is a risk of recurrence. In rare cases, prostatitis may result from cancer in the gland and so the cause should always be thoroughly investigated.

PROSTATE CANCER

Prostate cancer is a malignant condition of the prostate gland which, in its early stages, produces no or few symptoms and has consequently earned itself the dubious title of 'the silent killer'. Prostate cancer is the second most common form of malignancy in men, with over 12,000 new cases being identified each year. Most commonly, it is a cancer of older age with about half of new cases being identified in those aged over 75 years. In this older age group, the cancer tends to be slow-growing and it may not prove lethal within the normal life span of the individual. However, prostate cancer claims several thousand lives each year among men aged over 65 years and there is evidence that it is becoming more prevalent among younger age groups. Men aged 50 years and over are considered to be at risk but it is not unknown among those in their forties. Unfortunately, the disease appears to be more virulent in younger men but it is curable if it is caught and treated at an early stage.

Symptoms of prostate cancer may be few but when they do occur are similar to those of **BENIGN PROSTATIC HYPERTROPHY**. They include frequency of urination along with difficulty, discomfort and dull pain. These symptoms are much more likely to be caused by BPH than cancer but any man who is experiencing them must seek immediate medical help. All too often, a man does not report to his doctor because of embarrassment or fear but delay in treating this cancer can prove to be fatal. A doctor will be likely to examine the prostate gland by means of a digital rectal examination in order to detect any obvious growth. A further test may be carried out on a blood sample to detect a particular protein, prostate specific antigen (PSA), which often occurs at a high level in individuals with cancer. Further diagnostic tests using advanced scanning methods may be carried out to confirm the diagnosis.

Treatment methods depend upon individual circumstances, particularly the age of the patient and whether the cancer is the slow-growing form and has not spread. However, in many cases, **PROSTATECTOMY** (surgical excision of the prostate gland) will be needed or drug and hormone therapy to suppress the production of **ANDROGENS** which cause the tumour to grow. If the cancer has spread to other parts of the body, radiotherapy and/or chemotherapy may be required.

Cancer specialists have long complained that prostate cancer has been the 'Cinderella' among malignant diseases, attracting little funding for research or attention by the government and media. However, this situation is undergoing a change at the present time and there is now a great deal of discussion and published information about prostate cancer in the media in order to raise the level of awareness among men. In North America, men aged over 50 are encouraged to have a yearly rectal examination and PSA blood test to detect early cases of cancer. In the UK, there is debate about the overall usefulness of the PSA test as a screening technique as it is known that it can throw up false positives and equally, may sometimes fail to identify those with cancer. However, it seems certain that some sort of screening for men in the UK will be available in the near future. At the present time, individual men aged 50 and above may wish to discuss the screening options with their doctor.

Considerable research is being devoted to discovering preventative measures for prostate cancer in order to lessen the risks of contracting the disease but unfortunately, at the present time, most of this is experimental and some of it conflicting. However, it is suspected that both diet and environmental factors have a part in the prevention of cancer. Research has suggested that cooked tomatoes, tomato ketchup and foods containing selenium (nuts, e.g. Brazil nuts, egg yolks, seeds, whole grain cereals) and vitamin E may be protective. In general, a diet low in animal fat and high in vegetables and fruits, especially those with antioxidant properties (e.g. cranberries, blackberries, etc.) may be preventative and this is the diet recommended for general good health. Soya may also be protective. Promising new research results, centred on the cheap and widely available drug, aspirin, were recently announced in the UK. The results suggested that aspirin could combat existing prostate cancer and the drug may prove a useful tool in the treatment of the disease. Further research and clinical trials are expected to throw new light on these findings during the next few years.

PENIS

PHIMOSIS (TIGHT OR NON-RETRACTABLE FORESKIN)

Phimosis describes the condition in which the edge of the FORESKIN is narrowed and cannot be drawn back over the GLANS of the penis. It is a fairly common condition which usually becomes apparent during infancy or early childhood, although in some cases, it may arise as a result of infection in adult life. Typically, there is difficulty in passing urine with a poor stream or spraying because the opening is obstructed. There may be an increased risk of infections such as **BALANITIS**. Treatment invariably involves surgical removal of the foreskin, or circumcision, which is carried out under general anaesthetic. Pain-relieving drugs are needed to cope with post-operative pain which can be quite severe. However, the wound normally heals quite quickly although care is needed to minimize the risk of post-operative infection.

PARAPHIMOSIS

Paraphimosis is a condition in which the retracted foreskin becomes stuck or rolled up behind the glans penis and cannot be returned to its normal position. There is pain and swelling and the area may become gangrenous if not promptly treated. Treatment usually involves replacing the foreskin under general anaesthetic but circumcision may be performed to prevent recurrence.

BALANITIS AND RELATED INFECTIONS

Balanitis is inflammation and/or infection of the sensitive glans of the penis which results in itching, soreness, redness, heat and some swelling and discharge of pus (balanorrhagia) in severe cases. The usual cause is a bacterial or fungal infection which can be contracted indirectly as a result of **PHIMOSIS**. The condition is more common in childhood and sometimes occurs as a result of scratching, for instance if the boy is affected by eczema in the groin area. Occasionally, balanitis may be caused by an allergic reaction to a soap, detergent or some other agent, or infection may gain access because of poor personal hygiene. Treatment is usually by means of antibiotic or antifungal creams and possibly oral antibiotics, depending upon the cause. If the condition has arisen because of phimosis, circumcision is usually required.

BALANOPOSTHITIS

Balanoposthitis is a similar condition referring to a more generalized inflammation and infection of the glans penis and foreskin which causes pain, redness, irritation and discharge. It results from a bacterial or fungal infection and is treated by the application of appropriate creams and possibly other drugs.

BALANITIS XEROTICA OBLITERANS

Balanitis xerotica obliterans is a chronic skin disease of the penis in which a white, hardened area develops in the region surrounding the urethral opening. It is treated by application of antibacterial and anti-inflammatory ointments but in severe cases surgical treatment may be required.

CANCER OF THE PENIS

In the UK and other European countries, cancer of the penis is a rare cancer affecting about 1 in every 100,000 men, most commonly in those aged over 50 years. It usually appears as a small, painless rounded lesion or pimple but it may be concealed beneath the foreskin. If left, the lesion enlarges and begins to bleed or discharge and becomes painful. It may cause discomfort or pain on urination. The cancer spreads rapidly to lymph nodes in the groin and may then produce secondary tumours elsewhere in the body. If caught early, surgical removal of the tumour and foreskin may be sufficient but frequently, removal of part or all of the penis, along with local lymph nodes, is needed. Follow-up radiotherapy is then required.

Penile cancer does not occur in circumcised males and risk factors include poor personal hygiene and previous **BALANITIS XEROTICA OBLITERANS** and **ERYTHROPLASIA OF QYEYRAT**. Attention to personal cleanliness is important and uncircumcised males need to be particularly vigilant. Any unusual symptoms should always be reported to a doctor. This cancer can be successfully treated at an early stage.

ERYTHROPLASIA OF QYEYRAT

Erythroplasia of Qyeyrat is an uncommon, pre-malignant lesion which appears as a well-defined, reddish, soft patch on the glans penis. It is not capable of spreading beyond the local area and is treated by surgical removal and/or application of topical ointment containing fluoracil and possibly with other preparations also. Regular check-ups are then necessary as this condition increases the risk of the development of **CANCER OF THE PENIS**.

PRIAPISM

Priapism is a rare abnormality in which there is a persistent and painful erection of the penis which is not connected with sexual stimulation. The condition can be secondary to a number of conditions or infections or can be a side effect of several different types of drug. Priapism requires prompt medical intervention in order to prevent permanent damage to the tissues of the penis. It is an emergency condition which requires admittance to hospital and intervention to drain the blood away from the engorged tissues. Treatment is likely to be carried out under spinal or general anaesthetic and the underlying cause of the condition will require further investigation.

CHORDEE

Chordee is a congenital (i.e. present at birth) defect in which the penis is abnormally curved. It is caused by the presence of fibrous tissue next to the corpus spongiosum and may be associated with **HYPOSPADIAS**. It is usually treated by surgery during childhood.

HYPOSPADIAS

Hypospadias is a congenital defect in which the urethral opening is abnormally placed on the underside of the penis instead of at the tip. It is usually corrected by means of a surgical operation performed during early childhood.

EPISPADIAS

Epispadias is a congenital defect in which the urethral opening is abnormally placed on the upper side of the penis instead of at the tip. It is usually corrected by means of a surgical operation performed during early childhood.

PREVENTATIVE MEASURES FOR MEN

The male reproductive organs are subject to two main types of disorder – infections and cancer – and by ensuring that he is well-informed and self-aware, a man can reduce the risks that these conditions pose to his health. Traditionally, men in the UK have been far less likely to adopt measures to safeguard their health than women, although fortunately, attitudes are now changing. Where the genital and reproductive organs are concerned, embarrassment and fear remain major problems for men.

When women become sexually active and seek contraceptive advice, they enter a system which involves intimate gynaecological examination, the cervical smear test and discussion centred on sexual and reproductive health. Men escape all of this so that if problems arise, many are too embarrassed to even discuss them with their partner, never mind seeking help from the medical profession. A current advertising campaign, which seeks to address this issue, tells men 'Don't die of embarrassment' because it is undoubtedly the case that ignoring early symptoms and signs of cancer does and has cost lives.

SELF-EXAMINATION OF THE TESTICLES AND THE PENIS

The most important protective method for all men is to carry out regular self-examination of the testicles and penis.

This should begin around the age of 14 to 15 years and it is essential for parents to highlight the importance of this to their sons as part of any discussion on 'sex education'. Testicular self-examination should be carried out about once a month and the best time is following bathing or showering when the organs are warm and relaxed.

Use a mirror to become familiar with the normal size and appearance of the testicles. It is common for one to be slightly larger than the other but look out for any extra increase in size, weight or shape which might indicate abnormality. Use one hand to support the scrotum and with the fingers and thumb of the other, feel each testicle in turn. The small irregularities and bumps are all the highly coiled tubes of which each is largely composed. Familiarity with the normal texture, size, appearance and weight makes it more likely that any abnormality will be noticed. Likewise, any dull ache, sensation of heaviness or pain which persists for more than a few days should be reported to a doctor. The penis should also be examined. Any persistent sores, lesions or skin conditions require medical evaluation (*see also* **SEXUALLY TRANSMITTED DISEASES** and **SAFE SEX**).

As discussed above, disorders of the prostate gland are common in middle-aged and older men, particularly among those who are more than 50 years old. Benign prostatic hypertrophy is by far the most common and less serious disorder but cases of prostate cancer are also rising.

Prostate cancer produces no or few symptoms in its early stages but it can be detected by digital rectal examination and by blood tests. It is recommended that men aged over 50 should have a yearly rectal examination to detect possible cancer at an early stage when it can be successfully treated. By its nature, this procedure is difficult for many men to accept but other methods of detecting prostate cancer may become available in the future.

Men should also be aware that rarely, they can be affected by **BREAST CANCER** which is not solely a female disease. A lump in the region of the nipple or breast should always be evaluated medically in case of malignancy.

CHAPTER 4

The female reproductive system

The female reproductive organs comprise internal organs and structures, which include the ovaries, Fallopian tubes, uterus (womb) and vagina and the external structures of the vulva – the mons pubis, labia, clitoris and vaginal orifice.

THE ANATOMY OF THE FEMALE REPRODUCTIVE SYSTEM

The paired ovaries are the female gonads, i.e. the reproductive organs that produce the gametes (sex cells) or ova and important sex hormones. They are the direct equivalent of the male testicles. The ovaries are a pair of glands about the size and shape of almonds, situated in the upper part of the pelvic cavity on either side of the womb. Each ovary is surrounded by a protective, fibrous tissue capsule and is held in place by suspensory ligaments. The ovary is surrounded by a layer of germinal epithelium (a specialized tissue

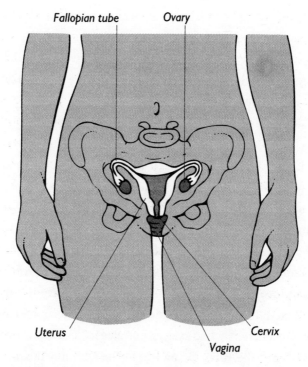

The female reproductive system

consisting of densely packed cells), giving way internally to connective tissue.

Housed within the connective tissue are numerous follicles which each consist of cells that nurture and surround an immature ovum (egg). Each ovary in a newborn baby girl contains about 70,000 primordial follicles containing primary oocytes or immature eggs. Only about 500 of these will eventually develop into

mature ova to be released during the woman's reproductive period between **PUBERTY** and the **MENOPAUSE**
(*see* **OOGENESIS**). The remainder form a pool of potential
gametes which are destined never to mature and which
eventually degenerate.

Each ovary lies in close proximity to a Fallopian tube
– a duct within the abdominal cavity. The paired
Fallopian tubes are about 10 to 12 cm long and each
extends from an ovary and loops downwards to
connect directly with the upper part of the uterus or
womb on either side. The upper part of each Fallopian
tube is expanded into a funnel-like structure, the
infundibulum, which forms a cup around the ovary.
Small projections called fimbriae extend from the
epithelial lining of the infundibulum and move to
create a current which sweeps a released egg from the
ovary into the tube. Below the infundibulum lies the
portion of the Fallopian tube known as the ampulla. It
is in this area that fertilization, the fusion of sperm and
egg, normally takes place. The Fallopian tubes descend
and connect directly with the upper part of the uterus
or womb, one on either side.

The uterus is a muscular, roughly pear-shaped organ
lying within the pelvic cavity between the bladder and
the rectum. This remarkable organ is only about 7.5
cm long and no more than 5 cm wide at its broadest
point, in its usual, unexpanded state. However, in the
event of pregnancy, it is capable of stretching and

expanding to support a foetus and placenta which weigh several kilograms, once fully formed. It is able to do this through a unique configuration of muscles – the myometrium – of which the bulk of the uterus is composed. Powerful contractions of the uterine muscles are able to expel the baby during labour.

The uterus is lined internally by a specialized, mucous membrane layer called the endometrium which has a plentiful blood supply. The endometrium undergoes a series of changes which make up the **MENSTRUAL CYCLE** and these coordinate with those that take place in the ovaries during the **OVARIAN CYCLE**. At its lower end, the uterus narrows to form a thinner neck or cervix which forms the connection with the lowest part of the female reproductive tract, the vagina. The cervix lies partly above and partly within the vagina, projecting into it and linking it with the cavity of the uterus via the cervical canal. The lining or epithelium of the cervix contains numerous small glands which secrete a lubricating cervical mucus, the consistency and viscosity of which alters in response to hormonal changes during the ovarian and menstrual cycles. The mucus is colourless and alkaline prior to the release of an egg but after ovulation, it becomes more copious and may be noticed as a clear or white discharge. It also becomes more acidic, which aids the survival of sperm and contains proteins and sugars which further sustain them. Deficiencies in cervical mucus can contribute towards **INFERTILITY** if the environment created is in some way hostile to the survival of sperm.

In the event of pregnancy, a further change occurs also under hormonal influence, with the formation of a thick mucus plug that blocks the cervical canal and prevents the passage of substances from the outside. Normally, the cervix is pink in colour but it turns bluish-purple in pregnancy because of an increase in its blood supply. This change, known as Chandwick's sign, is particularly pronounced during second and subsequent pregnancies. The lower end of the cervix exits into the vagina through an opening called the external os. In a woman who has never given birth, the diameter of the opening is about 5 mm. Following childbirth, it does not regain its former shape but becomes a slit about 7 mm long. During **LABOUR**, the cervix dilates greatly to a diameter of about 10 cm or more to allow for the passage of the baby into the birth canal.

The cervix opens into the vagina which is a relatively thin-walled, muscular passage that exits to the exterior through the vaginal orifice. It has muscular walls which are lined on the inside with mucous membrane and is capable of considerable expansion to allow for the passage of a baby during childbirth. The vagina receives the male penis during sexual intercourse and has a good supply of blood, making it capable of becoming firm and engorged during sexual arousal. Sperm are generally released fairly high up near to the cervix. The vagina is lubricated by cervical secretions and is the passage through which menstrual blood passes to the outside.

At birth, the vaginal orifice is protected on the inside by a thin membrane called the hymen. This usually tears to some extent as a girl grows older but may only be finally ruptured by first sexual intercourse. The external genitalia in the female are collectively known as the vulva and comprise the vaginal orifice, two pairs of skin folds – the labia minora and labia majora – the clitoris and the mons pubis (or veneris). The mons pubis is a pad of fatty tissue which overlies and protects the symphysis or central portion of the pelvic girdle bones. During **PUBERTY**, the covering skin grows pubic hair which forms a triangular pattern called the escutcheon.

The labia majora are two long folds of skin which are the equivalent of the scrotum in males. They extend from the mons pubis to the perineum (the area of skin, muscle and fibrous tissue between the anus and the vaginal orifice) and are well supplied with nerves and blood vessels which make them capable of enlargement during sexual arousal. They surround the labia minora, a pair of inner, thinner skin folds which extend around the clitoris to form a hood and protect the urethral and vaginal openings.

The clitoris is a small, cylindrical bulb of erectile tissue situated at the head of the labia minora above the urethral opening and beneath the pubic bone. It is the equivalent of the glans of the male penis and its only known function is for sexual pleasure. It is very sensitive and becomes engorged with blood during sexual stimulation and increases in size. It is the main focus for the production of orgasm in women. A pair of Bartholin's glands are located on either side of the vaginal orifice and these produce a mucus secretion during sexual arousal which has a lubricating function.

HORMONAL CONTROL AND THE OVARIAN CYCLE, MENSTRUAL CYCLE AND OOGENESIS

In contrast to males, in whom the production of sex cells and hormones is relatively constant, the female reproductive system is subject to a complex cyclical pattern of changes which affect both the ovaries and the womb. These changes are controlled by hormones which fluctuate in level – the fluctuations themselves being part of the control system through the operation of feedback loops. The cycles in the ovaries and womb are further coordinated with one another through the operation of these hormonal feedback loops. In non-pregnant women, the cycles last, on average, about 28 days but can vary greatly in duration between individuals. In the event of FERTILIZATION and the successful implantation of an embryo into the womb, the cycles are interrupted and a new system of hormonal control is implemented to sustain the **PREGNANCY**.

The primary female sex hormones are mainly produced by the ovaries and are called oestrogens and progesterone. Oestrogens are a group of steroid hormones which are additionally produced in small amounts by the adrenal glands, fatty tissues and placenta during pregnancy. At puberty, they are responsible for the development of the secondary sexual characteristics, the development of the female body shape with the laying down of additional fat and the maturation and growth of the reproductive organs. Throughout reproductive life, they play a vital role in the continuation of ovarian and menstrual cycles. Progesterone is also a steroid hormone whose main function is to prepare the endometrial lining of the womb to receive a fertilized egg. In the event of pregnancy, progesterone becomes even more important as it maintains the uterus and ensures that no further eggs are released from the ovaries. As pregnancy advances, the **PLACENTA** takes over from the ovaries as the main producer of progesterone. Synthetic oestrogens and progesterone are used in **CONTRACEPTION** and in **HORMONE REPLACEMENT THERAPY** (*see* **MENOPAUSE**).

As in the male, the production of the sex hormones in the female are stimulated by the release of other hormones from glands at the base of the brain. The hypothalamus secretes gonadotrophin-releasing hormone (GnRH) which acts on the anterior lobe of the pituitary gland – the adenohypophysis. The adeno-hypophysis produces and releases two hormones under the influence of GnRH – the gonadotrophins, Follicle-stimulating hormone (FSH) and luteinizing hormone (LH), respectively. Positive and negative feedback loops operate to regulate the ovarian and menstrual cycles through the fluctuating levels of the five hormones involved.

THE OVARIAN CYCLE

The ovarian cycle can be divided into three distinct phases. During the first, follicular phase, several folli-cles begin to grow in one ovary under the influence of FSH from the adenohypophysis. The immature folli-cles possess receptors for FSH but not for FH at this stage, although LH is being produced and released. Amounts of FSH and LH are low because oestrogen is also only being produced in small amounts. Although several follicles initially begin to grow, only one (or rarely two) continues to mature to become a roughly spherical-shaped Graafian follicle. This consists of an outer wall, composed of several layers of cells to which an egg cell or primary oocyte (*see* **OOGENESIS**) is attached at one point, surrounded by a fluid-filled cavity. The Graafian follicle becomes quite large and moves towards the surface of the ovary, forming a noticeable bulge. As the follicles grow and the follicular phase progresses, increasing amounts of oestrogen are produced (along with small quantities of **ANDROGENS** – the male hormones).

Receptors in the hypothalamus respond by releasing greater quantities of gonadotrophin-releasing hormone (GnRH) resulting, in turn, in a surge in the production of follicle-stimulating hormone (FSH) and luteinizing hormone (LH). The surge in LH is greater than that of FSH because the cells that produce this hormone in the pituitary become increasingly sensitive to GnRH at this time. Also the developing follicles have, by this stage, developed receptors which can detect and respond to LH. This LH sensitivity on the part of the follicles results in the final maturation of the one Graafian follicle while the others cease to develop and, as a result, oestrogen levels reach a plateau and then start to decline. The sharp increase in LH (and, to a lesser extent, FSH) closely follows the peak in oestrogen production, occurring within one or two days. The steep rise in the levels of oestrogen, LH and FSH, corresponding with the maturation of the Graafian follicle, brings the follicular phase to an end. This stage of the ovarian cycle is known as the ovulatory phase and ends with ovulation itself, which takes place about one day after the peak release of LH.

At ovulation, the surface of the Graafian follicle and the wall of the ovary burst open to release the egg

Section of the ovary showing ova in various stages of maturation.

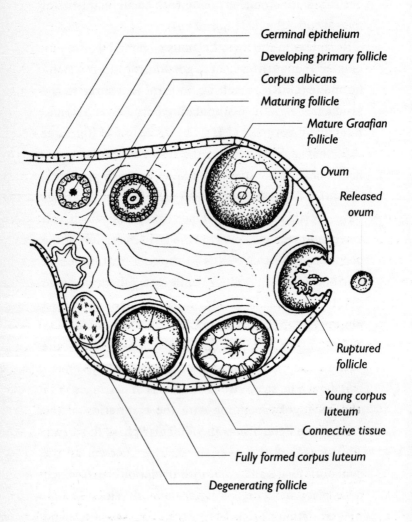

Germinal epithelium

Developing primary follicle

Corpus albicans

Maturing follicle

Mature Graafian follicle

Ovum

Released ovum

Ruptured follicle

Young corpus luteum

Connective tissue

Fully formed corpus luteum

Degenerating follicle

(secondary oocyte) which, at this stage, has not yet completed its development (*see* **OOGENESIS**). Following ovulation, the remaining tissue of the Graafian follicle has a further critical role to play. The tissues form a specialized, endocrine (i.e. hormone-producing) body or gland called the corpus luteum and the ovarian cycle enters the luteal phase which usually lasts for about 14 days. Although the LH level has peaked and has begun to decline, the amount is great enough to promote the corpus luteum to produce its hormones – progesterone and oestrogen. Output from the corpus luteum halts the decline in oestrogen levels – which now begin to rise again. The progesterone level increases even more sharply, overtaking that of oestrogen, with both reaching a plateau that corresponds with maximum activity in the corpus luteum.

Oestrogens and progesterone are responsible for preparing the lining of the womb for the reception and implantation of a fertilized egg. Progesterone has a critical part to play in the changes that take place within the womb and if pregnancy occurs it becomes the most important and essential hormone. The increasing concentrations of progesterone and oestrogen are interpreted by receptors in the hypothalamus, having an inhibitory effect on the release of GnRH. Hence the secretion of LH and FSH declines and eventually drops away quite steeply. The corpus luteum can only operate if LH is being produced. In the absence of LH, it starts to fail and eventually disintegrates and this, in turn, causes a sharp decline in the level of oestrogen, and progesterone ceases to be produced. The lowest point in these levels causes the onset of menstruation.

THE MENSTRUAL CYCLE

The menstrual cycle is also divided into three phases beginning with the menstrual flow phase during which bleeding or menstruation occurs. The onset of bleeding marks the first day of the cycle and, as mentioned above, it is triggered by low levels of progesterone and oestrogen as the corpus luteum in the ovary disintegrates. The blood vessels in the endometrium contract spasmodically, causing bleeding which usually occurs for a few days.

Then, under the influence of rising oestrogen production from the growing follicles in the ovary (ovarian follicular phase), the endometrium begins to thicken. This second stage of the menstrual cycle is called the proliferative phase during which time the tissues increase and a new blood supply begins to form. The endometrium and womb are being prepared for the possible reception of a fertilized egg, even though ovulation has not yet taken place in the ovary. After ovulation and stimulated by increasing levels of oestrogen and progesterone produced by the corpus luteum, the menstrual cycle enters the secretory phase.

The changes in hormone levels which take place, correlated with the ovarian and menstrual cycles along with a stylized view of the ovary.

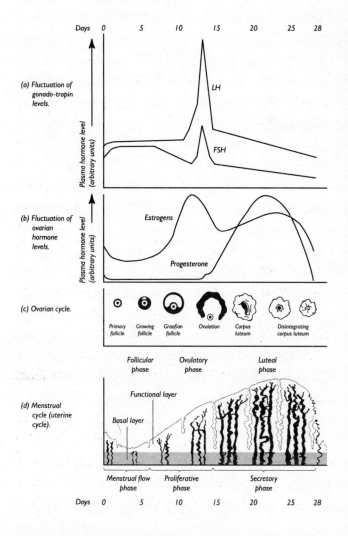

(a) Fluctuation of gonado-tropin levels.

Plasma hormone level (arbitrary units)

LH

FSH

(b) Fluctuation of ovarian hormone levels.

Plasma hormone level (arbitrary units)

Estrogens

Progesterone

(c) Ovarian cycle.

Primary follicle | Growing follicle | Graafian follicle | Ovulation | Corpus luteum | Disintegrating corpus luteum

Follicular phase | Ovulatory phase | Luteal phase

Functional layer

Basal layer

(d) Menstrual cycle (uterine cycle).

Menstrual flow phase | Proliferative phase | Secretory phase

Days 0 5 10 15 20 25 28

During this stage, which corresponds with the luteal phase in the ovary, the endometrium becomes even thicker and its blood supply increases. Also, glands within the endometrium enlarge and begin to produce secretions containing nutrients such as glycogen. These will nourish a developing embryo in the early stages following implantation, should pregnancy occur and this glandular activity occurs under the influence of progesterone produced by the corpus luteum. Eventually, after a period of roughly two weeks, the hormonal changes described above bring about the disintegration of the corpus luteum followed by the onset of bleeding at the start of another menstrual cycle. It is only in the event of pregnancy that the cyclical pattern is interrupted and new hormonal controls take over – changes which are briefly discussed in a later section.

An understanding of hormonal cycles, along with the ability to produce and utilize synthetic hormones, has enabled a wide range of medical treatments to be introduced which were impossible in the past (*see* **CONTRACEPTION, INFERTILITY AND ITS TREATMENT** and **HORMONE REPLACEMENT THERAPY**).

OOGENESIS

Oogenesis describes the process by which mature egg cells or ova are produced in the ovary which follows a different pattern of development than that of male

SPERMATGENESIS. Oogenesis begins well before birth in the ovaries of the female embryo. Precursor cells called primordial germ cells divide by the normal process of cell division (mitosis) to produce potential eggs known as oogonia (*sing.* oogonium). These cells are diploid, i.e. they contain the same full set of chromosomes as every other cell in the developing embryo.

Oogonia undergo many more mitotic divisions but finally enter the first phase of the specialized process of division called meiosis to produce primary oocytes which are still diploid. A baby girl is born with a full but finite number of primary oocytes which are all potential egg cells but only a very few are destined to mature. This is in contrast to spermatogenesis in which sperm cells are continually produced. The primary oocytes now enter long, resting phases although towards puberty, there is some development of the cells and their surrounding follicles.

After puberty, a few follicles develop in the ovary during each ovarian cycle in the manner described above. One primary oocyte then undergoes a further stage of division of the specialized process of meiosis. This produces a large secondary oocyte and a small by-product cell called the first polar body. It is the secondary oocyte which is shed on ovulation and the completion of meiosis only occurs if this cell is subsequently fertilized by a male sperm. In the event of fertilization taking place, the secondary oocyte completes meiosis by undertaking the second meiotic division. This produces a large haploid ootid which rapidly becomes a mature ovum and a second small polar body.

Hence, like the sperm, the ovum possesses half the number of chromosomes of every other parental cell, contained within a nucleus (a structure within each cell which houses genetic material). Up to four polar bodies may be produced during meiosis but all eventually disintegrate. The fact that oogenesis produces unequal cells after each division is again in striking contrast with spermatogenesis (*see* diagram).

During fertilization, the nuclei of sperm and egg unite, bringing together a new combination of chromosomes and thereby restoring a full diploid number which are unique to that individual.

Oogenesis

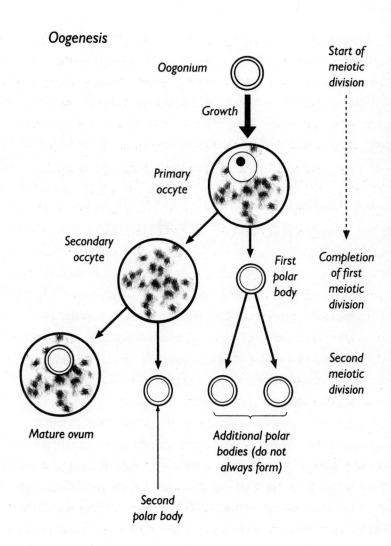

Oogonium

Growth

Primary oocyte

Secondary oocyte

First polar body

Mature ovum

Second polar body

Additional polar bodies (do not always form)

Start of meiotic division

Completion of first meiotic division

Second meiotic division

CHAPTER 5

Diseases and disorders of the female reproductive system and their treatment

The female reproductive organs and genitalia are subject to various diseases and disorders, some of which are more common than others. A familiarity with and understanding of these conditions should be essential knowledge for every young woman (and those concerned about her) from the time of puberty, so that she is better able to protect her health.

In this section, congenital, structural and cancerous disorders of the reproductive organs are described along with generalized infections which may be acquired by means other than sexual intimacy. **SEXUALLY TRANSMITTED DISEASES** are discussed in Chapter 11 of this book.

OVARIES
POLYCYSTIC OVARY SYNDROME
Polycystic ovary syndrome is a condition in which one

or both ovaries produce multiple, small cysts and recent screening has revealed that it is surprisingly common, affecting, to a greater or lesser degree, about 20 per cent of all women.

Many experience none, or perhaps only one or two of the characteristic symptoms which include infrequent or absent menstrual periods (amenorrhoea), weight gain or obesity and the appearance of masculine symptoms, particularly growth of hair on the face or chest (hirsutism) and acne.

The syndrome is thought to be caused by an imbalance in the production of pituitary hormones, with the result that the normally small output of **ANDROGENS** from the ovaries is increased. Treatment is usually hormonal, often in the form of the oral contraceptive pill and possibly other drugs to suppress androgen and counter the masculinizing effects. The condition can be psychologically distressing if the symptoms are marked but is not an illness, as such. Affected women may need hormones to stimulate the ovaries to release eggs if they wish to become pregnant.

OVARIAN CYST

Cysts that develop in the ovaries are usually benign but rarely, may be malignant. Cysts may occur singly in one ovary or more than one may develop in both ovaries. They are often 'functional', i.e. they may develop as a result of the normal functioning of the ovary. Hence, if a **GRAAFIAN FOLLICLE** fails, for some reason, to release its egg it may become a cyst as may a **CORPUS LUTEUM** that does not disintegrate normally.

Cysts vary in size and usually consist of a sac-like structure containing fluid or more solid material, attached to the ovary by means of a stalk. Functional cysts may disappear without producing symptoms and, in fact, ovarian cysts may remain undetected for this reason. If symptoms do arise, it is often because the cyst has become quite large and is impinging upon some other organ or because it is causing hormonal disturbance.

Hence the range of possible symptoms is quite wide and includes bloating in the lower abdomen, painful and frequent urination (if a cyst is affecting the bladder), disruption of the **MENSTRUAL CYCLE** or cessation of periods (amenorrhoea), pain with sexual intercourse, infertility, discoloured vaginal discharge and growth of facial and body hair (if excess androgens are being produced or female hormones are suppressed). In rare cases, the cyst may twist on its stalk causing extremely severe abdominal pain, high temperature and sickness and this is an emergency, requiring immediate hospital admittance and surgery.

Diagnosis of cysts is usually made by means of pelvic examination and ultrasound. Surgical treatment of a benign cyst is by means of laparoscopy to drain the structure and repair the ovary or, possibly, oophorectomy to remove the whole ovary. In the rare event of malignancy, it is necessary to remove the affected ovary and Fallopian tube. Further treatment will be needed if the disease has spread.

OVARIAN TUMOUR (BENIGN)

Ovarian tumours may be benign or malignant and both involve an abnormal growth of cells in an ovary. A benign tumour may resemble a CYST or it can occasionally grow huge to the extent of mimicking pregnancy. Symptoms produced by a benign tumour may be non-existent or they can be similar to those of an ovarian cyst. Also, the tumour may rarely twist and cause severe abdominal pain, fever and vomiting which requires immediate emergency surgery – usually removal of the affected ovary.

The tumour is diagnosed in much the same way as a cyst and evaluation will be made to decide on the best course of action. Hormonal treatment may be prescribed to shrink the tumour or, if not particularly troublesome, it may be left alone and monitored from time to time to see if it is changing in size. Ovarian tumours often disappear spontaneously but if symptoms are severe, surgical removal of the tumour and the ovary may be needed.

Provided that an unaffected ovary remains on the other side, normal conception and pregnancy can still take place although this may require a little more time.

OVARIAN TUMOUR (MALIGNANT)
OR CANCER OF THE OVARY

Ovarian cancer is a malignant growth of cells in one or both ovaries and women over the age of 40 are the most likely ones to be affected although the disease may strike at any age. Unfortunately, few or no symptoms are produced in the early stages when the cancer can be readily treated. Those that do occur include digestive upset and slight discomfort in the lower abdomen and irregular menstrual periods. These symptoms are all too often attributed to the onset of the menopause and so the tumour continues to grow, undetected. At a later stage, more pronounced symptoms may be produced including abdominal pain and the presence of a detectable mass, nausea, weight loss, digestive upsets, anaemia and painful sexual intercourse.

Diagnostic techniques include physical examination, ultrasound scan, blood tests and possibly biopsy by means of a laparoscopy (small incision in the abdomen) or culdotomy (needle extraction of cells through the blind end portion of the vagina which lies beneath the cervix). Treatment invariably involves surgical removal of the affected ovary (oophorectomy) and probably the Fallopian tube. The other ovary has to be checked very carefully and it may sometimes be necessary to remove it, along with its Fallopian tube and the womb (hysterectomy), if the cancer has spread. Radiotherapy and/or chemotherapy may also be required. Following initial treatment, and if surgical removal of both the ovaries and womb has been necessary, **HORMONE REPLACEMENT THERAPY** may be needed to relieve menopausal symptoms.

In recent years, ovarian cancer has deservedly received a great deal more attention, not only in terms of research into the cancer itself and into methods of early detection, but also into the development of new drugs and treatment regimes. The lack of early symptoms means that there is a considerable risk of the cancer spreading before it is detected and so developing reliable screening methods is vital in the fight against this disease. There appears to be a familial/genetic connection in some cases and so women who are at risk can already be screened by existing methods. New drugs and better treatment methods are improving survival times, even for women with more advanced cancer and there is the expectation that the situation will continue to improve in the future.

UTERUS OR WOMB
UTERINE POLYPS
Uterine polyps are soft growths of tissue, almost always benign, that may develop within the endometrium or lining of the womb. They may cause no symptoms at all or may be responsible for intermittent bleeding, especially after sexual intercourse. They may be

detected during a pelvic examination and, if trouble-some, may be removed by a **D AND C** or **HYSTEROSCOPY**. Polyps can recur but it is rare for them to become malignant.

D and C stands for dilation and curettage and it is one of the most common surgical gynaecological proce-dures, performed under general anaesthetic. The cervix is dilated and an instrument called a curette is passed through into the womb which is then used to remove part of the endometrium. D and C is used for diagnosis, as tissue can be obtained for biopsy (e.g. to look for **UTERINE CANCER** or to investigate **INFERTILITY**) but it is also a method of treatment.

Hence a D and C can be useful in correcting heavy menstrual bleeding (**MENORRHAGIA**), removing polyps and fibroids and is routinely performed following a miscarriage or female **STERILIZATION**. In addition, it is used to remove retained placental tissue which may be a complication of childbirth or abortion and uterine adhesions (scar tissue). Occasionally, it is used as a method of procuring an early abortion, if particular circumstances apply.

Hysteroscopy involves passing a special instrument called a hysteroscope into the cervical canal and uterus so that these can be examined visually. The instrument may then be used to provide the visual guide for removal of polyps by cauterization or surgery or retrieval of a 'lost' **INTRAUTERINE DEVICE** (IUD). Or the hysteroscope can be used to obtain a tissue sample for biopsy.

FIBROIDS (MYOMAS)

Fibroids are commonly occurring, almost always benign, tumours of the muscular wall of the uterus and consist of abnormal growths of muscle cells. They are much more common in Black women, for reasons that are not known, although there is evidence to suggest a hereditary, genetic connection in many cases. Fibroids are also more common in older women over the age of 35 but they do not develop after the menopause. Although there are several types of fibroid, they are often small (about the size of a pea) and frequently do not produce symptoms and remain undetected. More rarely, a fibroid may increase in size to the dimension of a large grapefruit and can weigh several kilograms.

If symptoms are produced, they very often relate to menstruation. Periods may be more frequent and often the flow is heavy enough to produce anaemia. Other symptoms include breakthrough bleeding between periods and pain and bleeding with sexual intercourse. If a fibroid is large and troublesome, it may press upon the bladder causing frequency of urination. Other possible symptoms are generalized lower abdominal pain or discomfort, depending upon the size and position of the fibroids and a more prolific vaginal discharge.

One possible consequence of fibroids is a decline in **FERTILITY,** as their presence may make it more difficult for a fertilized egg to become implanted in the womb. Also, fibroids may enlarge during pregnancy and possible affect the placenta or compromise the efficiency of the womb, increasing the risk of **MISCAR-RIAGE.**

Growth of fibroids is affected by the hormone **OESTROGEN** and in the event of a positive diagnosis, avoiding oral contraception may help to prevent enlargement or proliferation. Diagnosis of fibroids may be made from a pelvic examination, hysteroscopy or ultrasound scan along with reporting of symptoms. If menorrhagia (heavy bleeding) is the main symptom, a D and C procedure is often performed to confirm diagnosis and lessen the problem for a time. Other possible courses of action include endometrial resection and ablation – a relatively new procedure which involves removing almost all the endometrium by means of an electric current (diathermy) or laser beam. Alternatively, individual fibroids may be removed or, if the woman has no future desire to become pregnant, a hysterectomy may be considered.

In very rare cases (about 0.5 per cent) a fibroid may become malignant and, in this case, a hysterectomy may well be thought to be the best course of action to lessen the risk of spread of the cancer. However, following evaluation and if fibroids are benign and not too troublesome, as is often the case, it may be decided to leave them alone. After the MENOPAUSE, they invariably shrink and cause no further problems.

RETROVERTED AND RETROFLEXED UTERUS
A retroverted uterus is one which is tilted backwards in relation to the vagina. It may be congenital or arise after childbirth. A retroflexed uterus is one that is bent back on itself at an angle with the cervix. Menstrual cramps may be experienced in the lower back if the womb is in either of these positions and some women have greater difficulty in conceiving, but usually there are no problems. Occasionally it may be necessary to fit a vaginal pessary – a ring-shaped device which can help to support the uterus and bring it forwards.

PROLAPSED UTERUS
A uterus that has descended from its normal position so that it protrudes into the vagina or, in the most extreme cases, to the outside of the body. Slight prolapse is extremely common in women who have had children and may become more pronounced with advancing age as muscles become weaker. It only causes problems if it is pronounced, but a range of symptoms can be produced, depending upon the extent of the prolapse.

Symptoms include stress incontinence (a sudden involuntary release of urine as a result of an action that exerts pressure on the bladder, e.g. sneezing, coughing, laughing), backache, especially when lifting a heavy object, pelvic discomfort and possibly discomfort with urination and with sexual intercourse. The risk of developing or exacerbating a prolapsed uterus increases in those who are overweight or obese and with constipation and straining to move the bowels.

Treatment may not be necessary but occasionally a vaginal pessary can be fitted to support the cervix (*see* the section above on the **RETROVERTED UTERUS**). In more severe cases, a hysterectomy to surgically remove the womb may be the best course of action. **KEGEL EXERCISES** to strengthen the muscles of the pelvic floor are a self-help measure which can lessen the risk of a prolapse or prevent its further development (*see* the section on **PREVENTATIVE MEASURES** on page 93).

MENORRHAGIA (HEAVY BLEEDING)

Menorrhagia is a generalized term for menstruation that involves abnormally heavy or prolonged blood flow. Hence it includes women who have short menstrual cycles with bleeding every three weeks or less, those who bleed for perhaps seven days or longer or those who experience heavy bleeding lasting two or three days or more. Menorrhagia can result from fibroids, pelvic inflammation and infection, hormonal imbalance or presence of an intrauterine device (IUD). Excessive bleeding, whatever type of pattern it follows, usually results in anaemia with symptoms of fatigue, feeling cold, pallor and malaise. It occurs because the bone marrow cannot produce red blood cells quickly enough to replenish the steady, monthly loss and because it tends to arise over an extended time period, the woman may not realize that she is anaemic.

Fortunately, this type of anaemia can usually be readily treated by taking iron supplements. Correcting the menorrhagia itself depends upon the underlying cause which must first be ascertained and a D and C may well be performed as a diagnostic and treatment method. If the cause is hormonal, appropriate therapy might be the oral contraceptive pill or danazol – a synthetic androgen which suppresses the production of pituitary gland hormones. A relatively new treatment is the **PROGESTOGEN-RELEASING IUD** (*see* Chapter 10 on **CONTRACEPTION**) which makes bleeding very light or non-existent in women with menorrhagia which does not have an obvious cause. Other surgical treatments include endometrial resection and ablation (*see* **FIBROIDS**) and, possibly, a hysterectomy.

DYSMENORRHOEA (PAINFUL PERIODS)
Dysmenorrhoea is pain associated with menstrual periods and is commonly experienced to a certain extent by nearly all women at some stage during their

reproductive life. Uncomfortable cramp-like pains are experienced in the abdomen or lower back but usually these are fairly short-lived and can be relieved with ordinary analgesic drugs, a hot bath or hot water bottle. However, more severe symptoms are experienced by some women and it is to this condition that the term dysmenorrhoea is usually applied.

The condition can be primary, i.e. occurring within three years of menarche (the onset of menstruation) or secondary, arising at a later stage when there has been no previous history of problems. In both cases, the pain is severe and disabling, interfering with normal life and accompanied by other possible symptoms such as nausea, headache, vomiting, sweating, diarrhoea and malaise. Secondary dysmenorrhoea usually has an underlying cause such as the presence of FIBROIDS, an INTRAUTERINE DEVICE (IUD), PELVIC INFLAMMATORY DISEASE or ENDOMETRIOSIS. Hence treatment depends upon investigations to ascertain the underlying cause.

Both primary and secondary dysmenorrhoea involve hormones called prostaglandins which produce uterine contractions. Treatment is often hormonal – particularly the oral contraceptive pill which can be used to override the body's natural cycle and prevent the occurrence of disabling symptoms. A special form of IUD which releases progesterone may be recommended in some cases. Other pain-relieving drugs may also be prescribed, especially those such as ibuprofen and mefenamic acid which act as anti-prostaglandins.

ENDOMETRIOSIS

Endometriosis is a strange condition which is not a disorder of the uterus as such but involves material that originates from it, being caused by tissue derived from the endometrium growing abnormally outside the womb. The tissue usually attaches itself to the outer surfaces of organs in the lower abdomen and pelvic region including the womb itself, ovaries, Fallopian tubes and bowel or bladder. Rarely, it may even become deposited at sites farther away. The displaced tissue acts in exactly the same manner as it would if it were in situ in the womb, reacting to the hormonal changes of the menstrual cycle. Hence it thickens up and then is sloughed off, but cannot escape from the pelvic cavity and so floats freely until it becomes attached in its turn. Eventually the build-up may become so great that scar tissue and adhesions can form in which organs are abnormally joined together.

The cause is not fully established but it is believed that it arises from incomplete shedding of the thickened tissue lining of the womb during menstruation. It is thought that some of this tissue finds its way backwards up the Fallopian tubes and into the pelvic cavity where it floats and becomes attached, in the manner described above. Endometriosis is more common in young women aged between 20 and 30 but can occur at any time during the reproductive years. There is a greater risk of its development in those who never become pregnant. Pregnancy sometimes resolves or lessens the condition, which tends to become progressively more severe and threatens fertility. Women with endometriosis are advised to have children as soon as possible, if they wish to have a family at all. Endometriosis does, however, subside after the MENOPAUSE but older women who have completed their family may be advised to have all the internal reproductive organs (womb, ovaries and Fallopian tubes) surgically removed in order to resolve the condition.

Symptoms include pain that can be severe (DYSMEN-ORRHOEA) during menstruation but which becomes more acute towards the end of the period of bleeding. Also, pain during sexual intercourse and sometimes during urination (dysuria) or bowel movements. Blood may be present in the urine and occasionally on faeces and more generalized lower abdominal pain may occur, especially if adhesions have formed internally. There is a risk of INFERTILITY if implanted tissues block the Fallopian tubes. Endometriosis can be difficult to diagnose and may involve exploratory procedures such as laparoscopy. Hormonal treatments such as oral contraceptives may help or danazol, a synthetic androgen which inhibits the production of pituitary gland hormones. Surgery may be needed to free adhesions, or to attempt to unblock the Fallopian tubes or, more radically, to remove the internal reproductive organs. Women with endometriosis may require medical intervention or assistance before they can conceive, particularly if the condition has been present for some time.

ENDOMETRITIS

Endometritis is inflammation and infection of the endometrium producing symptoms of pelvic pain, fever, a vaginal discharge which may be foul smelling and a tender uterus. The cause may be irritation and infection from an **INTRAUTERINE DEVICE** or following abortion or childbirth. The infection is usually bacterial and is treated with appropriate courses of antibiotics and removal of an IUD, if present.

CERVIX

CERVICAL POLYP

A cervical polyp is the same as the polyps which sometimes grow in the main body of the womb, namely a small, fleshy, tear-shaped growth which is almost always benign. Polyps develop from the membranous lining of the cervix and are usually found high up in the cervical canal near the entrance to the womb. They may occur singly or in groups and may or may not give rise to symptoms which include cramping pain, bleeding after sexual intercourse and between menstrual periods. Polyps are usually readily detected and can be removed using cauterization techniques.

CERVICITIS

Cervicitis describes inflammation of the cervix which is often caused by infection. Inflammation alone can be caused by sexual intercourse, a spermicidal preparation or irritation from a foreign body such as the string of an **INTRAUTERINE DEVICE**, a condom or presence of a tampon. When infection is also present, a common cause is a **SEXUALLY TRANSMITTED DISEASE** but occasionally, it is of undiagnosed origin. Symptoms include pelvic pain, copious vaginal discharge, pain during intercourse and unexpected bleeding. However, the condition varies in severity and treatment depends upon the underlying cause. It may resolve without treatment or require courses of antibiotics or, more rarely, surgical intervention, in severe and persistent cases.

CERVICAL EROSION

Cervical erosion is a condition in which an abnormal area of epithelial lining develops at the end of the cervix – usually as an extension of tissue from the womb itself. The condition may arise as a result of trauma or damage in **CHILDBIRTH**, **ABORTION** or **MISCARRIAGE**, occur during **PREGNANCY** or result from the use of the **CONTRACEPTIVE PILL** or be of unknown origin. Symptoms are often not present, but occasionally, a more copious vaginal discharge or unexplained bleeding may occur. Treatment may not be necessary but can involve cauterization of the abnormal tissue. Rarely, erosion may indicate precancerous changes (*see* **DYSPLASIA, CERVICAL INTRA-EPITHELIAL NEOPLASIA AND CERVICAL CANCER**).

CERVICAL EVERSION
Cervical eversion is a condition resulting from trauma during **CHILDBIRTH** in which the cervix is damaged and the edge turns outwards.

INCOMPETENT CERVIX
Incompetent cervix is a rare condition arising in **PREGNANCY**, in which the cervix becomes fully dilated before gestation is complete. It frequently occurs around the 3rd or 4th month, resulting in rupture of the amniotic membranes and **MISCARRIAGE**. It may be the product of an earlier injury to the cervix, usually caused during a previous delivery which has resulted in weakness. Also, women who were exposed to diethylstilboestrol during foetal development have a high incidence of this condition. A woman may experience one or more **MISCARRIAGES** before the condition is diagnosed. In a subsequent pregnancy, the cervix may require to be sutured (stitched) to keep it closed, the

stitches being removed shortly before the expected date of delivery.

DYSPLASIA, CERVICAL INTRA-EPITHELIAL NEOPLASIA AND CERVICAL CANCER

Dysplasia means any abnormal development of cells and tissues and it is a term which is often used in reference to changes in the cells of the cervix which may indicate a precancerous state. The epithelial lining of the cervix consists of several layers that are constantly growing to renew ageing cells. New cells grow in the basal layer and move towards the surface, maturing as they do so. When precancerous changes or dysplasia occurs, the process is disrupted and the cells may appear to be abnormal or unusual or occur in places where they are not expected.

Cervical intra-epithelial neoplasia or CIN is a method of grading the changes in the cervical cells. CIN 1 is mild dysplasia; CIN 2 is moderate dysplasia and CIN 3 is severe dysplasia, also defined as being cancer in situ. This state defines cancer which is localized, and has not invaded surrounding tissues. CIN 1 and 2 are precancerous stages. Cervical dysplasia may cause the appearance of the cervix to change; there may be white patches (leucoplakia) or raised, red areas. The cells are sampled by means of a **CERVICAL SMEAR TEST** for microscopic examination in a laboratory. If dysplasia is discovered, further investigation is carried out. Usually, this involves a close examination of the cervix using an instrument called a colposcope which is inserted into the vagina.

Colposcopy is a simple procedure, lasting about 15 or 20 minutes and enables an evaluation to be made and possibly, a biopsy of the unusual area to be obtained. The dysplasia may be treated by cryosurgery (freezing), cauterization (heat) or laser surgery which destroys the abnormal cells. However, dysplasia may recur and since it usually produces no symptoms, it emphasizes the importance for women of the cervical smear test.

Causes of dysplasia are usually unknown but risk factors include early and frequent sexual intercourse during the teenage years, many sexual partners, infections of the reproductive tract, repeated pregnancies and smoking.

Cervical cancer is an abnormal growth of malignant cells in the cervix which may arise in two forms. Adenocarcinoma occurs in the epithelium of the cervical canal and squamous carcinoma affects the surface epithelium. Both types are invasive and capable of spreading beyond the womb but they are also detectable with the cervical smear test and can be successfully treated if caught at an early stage. Symptoms, which are only produced at a more advanced stage, include unexpected vaginal bleeding, e.g. between menstrual periods or after intercourse and also, post-menopausal bleeding, vaginal discharge, pain in the lower abdomen, unexplained weight loss, anaemia, loss of appetite and general malaise.

Diagnosis is usually made via an abnormal cervical smear which prompts further investigation such as colposcopy, or **CONE BIOPSY**. Cone biopsy is a surgical procedure carried out under a general anaesthetic, in which a cone-shaped section of cervical tissue is removed for microscopic examination. It may also be used as a treatment method for dysplasia or early cancer of the cervix and can be sufficient to remove the patch of suspect cells. A woman who has a cone biopsy is likely to experience some post-operative bleeding but occasionally, there can be other complications. A cone biopsy narrows the cervical canal and this may reduce fertility and the production of mucus may also be impeded. The surgery may give rise to **CERVICAL INCOMPETENCE** hence increasing the risk of **MISCARRIAGE** in the event of **PREGNANCY**.

Due to these potential problems, **COLPOSCOPY** is normally used in preference to cone biopsy as a diagnostic method. Treatment then involves relatively minor surgery such as cryosurgery, cauterization or laser surgery to remove the affected area. More advanced cancer may require more radical surgery to remove the diseased organs – usually hysterectomy – and possibly other affected tissues. Follow-up radio-therapy and/or chemotherapy may then be needed.

The prognosis is extremely good for early cervical

cancer and even at a more advanced stage, provided that the disease has not spread to other organs, the outcome can be favourable. This is a common female cancer but regular cervical screening offers the chance of early detection and a complete cure. Risk factors for cervical cancer are the same as those for dysplasia.

PELVIC INFLAMMATORY DISEASE (PID)

Pelvic inflammatory disease (PID) can affect the Fallopian tubes, ovaries and uterus and is the result of bacterial infection, but **CHLAMYDIA** and **GONORRHOEA** are responsible for many cases. Escherichia coli and the tuberculosis bacterium can also cause PID. The disease can be acute or chronic. Acute PID causes severe abdominal pain, high fever, chills, foul-smelling vaginal discharge and abdominal tenderness. Frequently adhesions form between the pelvic organs and the intestines or rectum which can be extremely painful. A pelvic examination and laboratory analysis of the discharge aid diagnosis.

A complication in both acute and chronic PID is the formation of an abscess that may need surgical drainage. If it bursts, such an abscess can cause infection of the entire pelvic and abdominal cavity. Blood poisoning or the filling of a Fallopian tube with fluid that may cause it to burst, are other possible complications of acute PID. However, these complications are rare as the severe pain brought about by acute PID usually causes most women to seek prompt medical attention.

Treatment is by means of antibiotics and bed rest. The condition usually improves within 2 weeks but, if not, another antibiotic is given. If 3 courses of antibiotics do not clear the infection, then the disease is deemed to have become chronic. Chronic PID results in a low level of infection that can continue for weeks or months.

Symptoms are persistent abdominal pain or cramps, fatigue, weakness and very heavy menstrual periods. Some mild cases have few or no symptoms but can cause partial or total infertility. Even in a mild form, adhesions may form and distort the Fallopian tubes, changing their shape or sealing their open end, so affecting fertility. Partial blockage of a tube leads to a higher risk of an ECTOPIC PREGNANCY, and the scar tissue can cause severe pain during sexual intercourse and menstrual periods.

Some case of PID respond well to bed rest and oral antibiotics, and severe infections may only be resolved by surgery to remove adhesions, or even the reproductive organs.

The use of an intrauterine device increases the risk of contracting pelvic inflammatory disease as does a D and C, abortion, or delivery of a baby. The use of condoms and diaphragms helps prevent the spread of this and all sexually transmitted diseases. PID can recur and any abnormal vaginal discharge should always be investigated.

A cervical smear test (Pap test) is a simple, painless procedure carried out to detect precancerous and cancerous changes in the cells of the cervix. A speculum is inserted into the vagina and cervical cells are sampled using a spatula or swab and these are then transferred to a glass slide for microscopic examination. The slides are sent to a hospital laboratory where they are examined by trained medical technicians who are expert in detecting anomalies. Results are normally available within about 6 weeks. If an unusual result is obtained, the woman is notified and asked to have another smear test to see if the change is still present. If this is the case, she will usually be advised to have a further investigation such as a **COLPOSCOPY**, normally carried out in hospital. It should be emphasized that an anomalous result does not necessarily indicate a precancerous condition. Undiagnosed infections or other factors can cause changes in cervical cells.

The cervical smear test should be undertaken every three years from the age of 18, or from the time when a young woman becomes sexually active. Recall letters for repeat screenings are routinely sent out to most women who are registered with GPs in the UK. However, it is up to each individual to ensure that she presents herself for the test, which remains the best method of detecting and hence treating this particular form of cancer at an early and curable stage.

VAGINA

VAGINITIS (NON-SPECIFIC, THRUSH, POST-MENOPAUSAL AND HORMONAL)

Vaginitis is inflammation of the vagina and vulva resulting in severe itching and heat and often accompanied by an abnormal discharge and infection. Vaginitis can accompany a **SEXUALLY TRANSMITTED DISEASE** but opportunistic infections can also cause the condition and it is these that are discussed here.

Non-specific vaginitis causes the symptoms listed above along with a vaginal discharge that smells unpleasant. It is caused by one of a number of organisms that normally inhabit the area of the vagina and rectum, without causing harm, such as Gardnerella and Escherichia coli. (E. coli is a natural inhabitant of the digestive tract but it commonly finds its way into the vagina.) These organisms can be responsible for infections if certain conditions arise. These include lowered immunity and poor health, hormonal disruption, development of diabetes mellitus and a change in the local environment of the vagina. The latter may arise during hot weather when there is increased sweating, especially if the woman is obese or is wearing underwear made of non-breathable material. Also, if there is a hormonal imbalance, of which the most common cause is the **MENOPAUSE**, the pH (degree of acidity or alkalinity) of the vagina changes and there is a decrease in the production of natural secretions.

Post-menopausal or atrophic vaginitis is quite common during or just after the menopause. Lowered immunity which decreases resistance to infection, often accompanies illness or its treatment, for example, radiotherapy or chemotherapy for cancer. In these circumstances, vaginitis may occur as an opportunistic infection caused by one of the organisms mentioned above or by the yeast-like organisms, Candida albicans or Monilia which are responsible for thrush. Yeast infections are responsible for about half of all the cases of vaginitis, producing itching, redness and a thick, whitish discharge that resembles cottage cheese. The causal organisms live in the vagina where they are usually kept at low levels by the normal acidic environment. However, if the acidic balance is upset, the yeasts may multiply and cause a thrush infection. Hormonal disruption as in **PREGNANCY** or taking oral contraceptives may be the trigger but also, courses of some antibiotics may alter the pH of the vagina. Other causes are those previously listed, i.e. ill-health and suppressed immunity, diabetes mellitus, hot weather with increased sweating, obesity and wearing non-breathable, close fitting underwear.

Treatment for vaginitis depends upon its cause and may require a course of antibiotics or anti-fungal drugs. These are often administered by means of vaginal creams and pessaries. To prevent reinfection if thrush or Gardnerella infection (also called bacterial vaginosis or BV) is diagnosed, male partners should also be given appropriate treatment in the form of a cream to apply to the penis.

Preventative measures include losing weight if obese, wearing underwear made of natural, rather than synthetic, fibres and avoiding tight-fitting clothes, attention to personal hygiene and wiping from front to back after using the toilet. HORMONE REPLACEMENT THERAPY may help post-menopausal vaginitis by restoring the body's lost oestrogen as may local application of oestrogen-containing creams or suppositories.

VAGINAL ATROPHY

Vaginal atrophy is a condition which affects older women after the MENOPAUSE in which there is a thinning of the tissues that line the vaginal walls and dryness due to a decrease in natural secretions. It is caused by a loss of oestrogen and a woman may experience discomfort or pain during intercourse and be more susceptible to infections of the reproductive and urinary tracts. The use of simple, lubricating gels and pessaries can ease the condition, and HORMONE RELACEMENT THERAPY to restore oestrogen is often beneficial.

UNEXPECTED VAGINAL BLEEDING

Any bleeding outwith normal menstruation can have a variety of different causes and needs to be investigated. CERVICAL EROSION, CYSTS, POLYPS, FIBROIDS, hormonal imbalance, infection, trauma or injury to the reproductive tract, ECTOPIC PREGNANCY and CANCER are all possible causes. Bleeding during PREGNANCY should always be reported as it may indicate a risk of MISCARRIAGE. Breakthrough bleeding may arise in a woman who has recently started taking oral contraception and it usually indicates that the dose is not suitable for the individual concerned.

Treatment of abnormal bleeding depends upon cause and investigation to establish this may involve a D and C or some other technique to eliminate the possibility of cancer.

VAGINAL CANCER

Vaginal cancer is an abnormal growth of malignant cells in the tissues of the vagina and/or vulva. This is usually a rare cancer but has been common in the daughters of women who took diethylstilboestrol (DES) during pregnancy. DES is a synthetic oestrogen which was prescribed until 1971 as a preventative against early MISCARRIAGE. It was given to women who had a history of miscarriage but has proved to have had a damaging effect on both mothers and their female children. Daughters have developed a particular form of vaginal cancer, clear-cell adenocarcinoma and also adenosis, an abnormal growth of glandular tissue in the vagina and cervix which is believed to be a precancerous condition.

Treatment of vaginal cancer usually requires surgery and radiotherapy but there is a risk that it may spread to other pelvic organs or beyond.

CYSTOCELE, URETHROCELE AND RECTOCELE

A cystocele is a prolapse at the base of the bladder in which it bulges into the vaginal canal. A urethrocele is a protrusion of the urethra into the vagina and it frequently accompanies cystocele. A rectocele is a prolapse of the wall of the rectum into the vagina which may occur with cystocele and a prolapsed uterus.

All these conditions usually arise due to a weakening of the pelvic floor muscles as a result of childbirth but may not manifest themselves until older age. **PELVIC FLOOR EXERCISES** or **KEGEL EXERCISES** to strengthen the muscles of the pelvic floor can help to prevent a prolapse and the conditions may be corrected with minor surgery if necessary.

GENITAL ITCHING OR PRURITIS VULVAE

Genital itching or pruritis vulvae consists of severe itching of the skin and tissues in the genital and anal region which can have a variety of causes. Common causes are **THRUSH** or other vaginal infections, hormonal imbalance especially at the time of the **MENOPAUSE,** allergic reaction to a soap, bath or shower product and untreated diabetes mellitus. Pubic or crab lice are insect parasites that can affect those having to live in insanitary conditions without access to washing facilities. They live among pubic hair and feed by sucking a minute amount of blood, laying numerous eggs (nits) during their 30-day life span.

Pubic lice cause intense itching and irritation and can be acquired from infected clothing or bedding and via sexual intercourse with an infected partner. They can affect both women and men but are readily treatable by the application of insecticidal preparations such as Malathion™. All members of a family or household should receive treatment. Infected clothing and bedding should either be burnt or thoroughly washed in the hot cycle of a washing machine and then ironed to ensure that all the lice and their eggs are destroyed.

PREVENTATIVE MEASURES FOR WOMEN

The female reproductive organs are subject to two main types of disorder – infections and cancer – and by ensuring that she is well-informed and self-aware, a woman can reduce the risks that these conditions pose to her health. The most important preventative measure for women is the **CERVICAL SMEAR TEST** which is carried out every three years. An examination of the pelvic organs may be carried out at the same time. This test identifies precancerous changes at an early stage when treatment is relatively simple and entirely successful. It is widely regarded as one of the best universal screening methods available and so it is important for every woman to make an appointment to have the test when she is asked to do so.

Other than this, the most important protective measure involves common sense and avoidance of known risk factors along with prompt reporting of any adverse or abnormal symptoms. Known risk factors for women include becoming sexually active at an early age, having numerous sexual partners and having unprotected sex.

Good personal hygiene is important but the chemicals used in scented soaps, bath and shower products or 'feminine deodorants' can cause irritation of the genital tissues in susceptible people. It is best to use a good quality soap and plain warm water and to avoid over-washing of the genital region. Vaginal douching, that is introducing warm water into the vagina, should be avoided unless it is undertaken on medical advice as treatment for a particular disorder. Unusual symptoms that should always be reported include abnormal bleeding, a discharge that smells offensive and pain. The sooner the cause of such symptoms can be established, the greater the likelihood of successful treatment.

PELVIC FLOOR OR KEGEL EXERCISES

Pelvic floor or Kegel exercises are a simple set of exercises to tone the muscles of the pelvic floor after childbirth. The muscles should be alternately contracted, 'held' for a count of five and then relaxed and the exercise repeated as many time a day as possible. The best way of locating the muscles involved is to try and stop the flow of urine while using the toilet. Usually, the anal muscles are contracted at the same time but it is possible to become aware of the operation of the vaginal muscles by this method.

These exercises are highly useful in preventing the development of a prolapse and can be easily performed and practised at any time. They can greatly improve the situation, even when a slight prolapse is present and also increase sexual enjoyment by enhancing the muscular tone of the vagina. Although it may seem difficult to perform the exercises in the days immediately following childbirth, or at a later stage when the muscles may have become slack, it is well worth the effort.

CHAPTER 6

The breasts

The breasts are not part of the reproductive system as such, since their primary function is to produce milk to feed an infant. However, they are important in female sexuality and self-image and are generally regarded as part of a woman's sexual apparatus.

STRUCTURE AND FUNCTION OF THE BREAST

Each breast is a compound mammary gland composed of milk-producing cells and ducts surrounded by fatty tissue and ligaments, all richly supplied by blood and lymph vessels. The milk-producing glands or acini are contained in discreet areas called lobules which are separated from one another by supporting fibrous and fatty tissue. Milk produced in a lobule passes into a duct which drains forwards towards the front of the breast. The ducts eventually unite to form about 15 to 20 larger ducts which each discharge milk through a separate opening in the nipple. Behind the nipple, the large ducts are expanded in places to form reservoirs called ampullae where milk is stored prior to discharge. The presence of milk-producing glands, fatty tissue and ligaments make the breasts feel as thought they are full of small lumps when the skin is pressed and this is entirely normal.

Nipples vary in size and have tiny muscles at the base which, when contracted, enable them to become erect – a response which occurs during sexual arousal. Each nipple is surrounded by a darker pigmented area called the areola. Each breast lies partly over the ribs, extending from the 2nd or 3rd down to the 5th or 6th on either side and partly over the pectoral muscles of the upper chest. A tail of breast tissue reaches into each armpit, containing lymph vessels which drain into lymph nodes under the arm. If breast cancer is present and begins to spread, the lymph nodes in the armpit are one of the first sites to be affected.

A foetus shows the first signs of breast development at about six weeks of GESTATION. Both male and female foetuses develop a line of primitive nipples over an area extending from the groin to the arm bud but over the next three weeks, all are reabsorbed apart from two which remain in the expected position on the chest. In the female foetus, the milk ducts begin to develop at about 12 weeks gestation but then there is no more growth until PUBERTY. The release of oestrogen at puberty causes elongation and branching of the existing milk ducts and laying down of fatty and connective tissue so that the breasts swell. The areola develops and darkens and progesterone release stimulates the development of the milk-producing cells and glands – a process which continues into early adulthood.

DISEASES AND CONDITIONS OF THE BREAST AND THEIR TREATMENT

The breast can be affected by a variety of different disorders, most of which are characterized by the development of lumps. There is a confusing array of medical names used to describe breast lumps and sometimes, the same term may be used in different ways. Discovery of a breast lump inevitably causes a great deal of stress, with most women immediately fearing that they have cancer. It is important to remember that the great majority of breast lumps are benign and even when this is not the case, the outlook for women with cancer is better now than at any time in the past and continues to improve.

BENIGN BREAST LUMPS
Fibroadenoma

Fibroadenoma is the commonest type of benign breast lump, mainly affecting young women in the 15 to 35 age range and usually occurring as two to four small tumours, possibly in both breasts. A fibroadenoma is firm, rubbery and smooth with well-defined edges and is composed of connective and glandular tissue. A biopsy is usually required to confirm the nature of the lump which may then be surgically removed. In some cases, hormonal drug treatments may be tried but these must be used cautiously. Fibroadenomas often recur so a woman with a history of this condition should be vigilant about **BREAST SELF-EXAMINATION**. Medical monitoring may be appropriate in some cases. Rarely, a fibroadenoma can develop into a form of non-invasive cancer but this can be readily treated.

Other fibrous breast lumps

Other fibrous breast lumps usually affect older women in the pre- and post-menopausal age range as this is the period when natural changes take place within the breast. More specifically, fatty tissue and milk-producing glands are increasingly replaced by fibrous connective tissue which may form poorly defined, firm lumps. Once diagnosis has been confirmed, there is no need for further treatment as surgery is difficult and this condition is always benign.

Hardened milk glands
(sclerosing adenosis)

Hardened milk glands or sclerosing adenosis is a condition in which a milk-producing gland enlarges and hardens producing a firm, ill-defined lump which is sometimes painful. Pain may be experienced if the lump is felt and also tends to occur before the onset of a period. Once again, this condition usually affects older women but is not unknown in younger ones and treatment is by means of surgical removal.

Breast cyst

A breast cyst is an accumulation of fluid that forms inside a milk duct or lobule and it is initially soft and undetectable. The fluid may vary in colour from cloudy or yellow-green to grey, brown or nearly black depending upon its constituents, which include proteins, hormones and lymph. A cyst may be very small or quite large, up to 5 cm in diameter, in which case it is clearly visible and may be hard. Cysts may also occur in clusters and usually affect the upper part of the breast.

If the amount of fluid inside the cyst increases or there is leakage, intense pain may be experienced and some fluid may exude from the nipples. The pain is caused by increased pressure and a woman may be unaware of the presence of the cyst until it becomes painful.

Treatment is by means of aspiration – withdrawal of the fluid through a fine needle – and the contents of the cyst may be sent for laboratory analysis if blood is present to make absolutely sure that there is no malignancy. Cysts are, however, benign and they are most common between the ages of 35 and 50 but do not arise after the MENOPAUSE, even in a woman who has a previous history of occurrence. For this reason, it is believed that the development of cysts is linked with high hormone levels, almost certainly oestrogen. However, hormone treatments are generally deemed inappropriate since a cyst is usually a one-off development and recurrence is uncommon. In the event of recurrence, the same cyst may refill again or another may appear elsewhere and aspiration is then repeated.

Galactocoele

A galactocoele is a cyst that is, in fact, a blocked milk duct and is smooth, soft and easily moved. It affects women who have recently been breast-feeding or who have given birth and produced milk and usually arises close to the nipple. It occurs most commonly if breast feeding is suddenly stopped or if drug treatments are given to halt the production of milk. The cyst can be aspirated if necessary and usually there are no further problems.

Intraductal papilloma

An intraductal papilloma is an uncommon, small, wart-like and usually benign growth which arises in one of the major milk ducts that open into the nipple. Papilloma most commonly affects women in their forties and causes a discharge from the nipple which may contain blood. Occasionally, there may be tenderness or slight pain caused by the pressure of the fluid in the duct. Single papillomas are almost always removed surgically for laboratory analysis as they can rarely be malignant. If more than one papilloma is present, the risk of malignancy is somewhat increased and the whole of the affected duct is removed. A woman who has been treated for intraductal papilloma should receive regular breast check-ups as the condition may recur.

Lipomas

Lipomas are non-malignant soft lumps composed of fat which are visible beneath the skin and can develop anywhere in the body and not particularly in the breast. However, if a lipoma occurs in the breast, it will warrant investigation because it may resemble a cancerous growth. Mammography will usually identify the lipoma for what it is and it is usually then left alone, unless its presence is causing significant problems.

Fat necrosis

Fat necrosis is a very rare response to a blow or injury to the breast which was severe enough to cause bruising and rupture of fat cells. The fat that is released from the cells may be treated as foreign material by the body's immune system and become sealed with scar tissue, forming a solid and irregular lump. Depending upon the age of the woman, the sealed fat may be hard and white (in the elderly) or softer and more oily (in younger age groups). Since the condition can resemble breast cancer, mammography, possibly followed by surgical removal, will be required but this is an entirely benign condition.

BREAST INFECTIONS

In general, infections of the breast are rare except during **BREASTFEEDING** and when they do occur, they are usually caused by bacteria that live on the skin. These bacteria may gain access via an abrasion on the nipple, usually a love-bite, enabling an opportunistic infection to occur. Signs of infection include redness, heat, swelling, pain, fever and malaise. If left untreated, an abscess filled with pus will develop and ripen and this is characterized by throbbing pain and fever.

Early signs of infection should not be ignored but immediately reported to a doctor who will prescribe appropriate antibiotics. These may be enough to prevent the full development of an abscess, and rest and the use of over-the-counter pain killers will also help to counteract other symptoms. However, if an abscess does develop it may need to be dealt with surgically, along with antibiotics to eliminate the infection (*see also* **BREASTFEEDING**).

Mammary duct ectasia

Mammary duct ectasia is a benign condition in which

ducts in the breasts dilate and become clogged with a thick fluid that may be cream, brown or green in colour. Symptoms include nipple discharge with leakage of some of the fluid from the ducts, strange-shaped lumps, burning pain and itching and possibly swelling and infection. The discharge may occasion-ally be streaked with blood and the affected ducts are often those closest to the nipple. The accumulation of fluid and waste products readily causes inflammation and easy access for infection. Ulceration or the forma-tion of an abscess may follow and inflammation of the ducts and surrounding tissue may cause scar tissue to be produced. Scar tissue may then harden and contract and pull upon the nipple, causing it to flatten or invert and, if this occurs, it must always be investigated to eliminate any possibility of cancer.

The condition may resolve on its own but inflamma-tion and infection must be treated with antibiotics. The fluid can be aspirated but there is a risk that it may return. In severe cases, a surgical operation to remove the affected ducts may be required.

MASTALGIA

Mastalgia is breast pain, often accompanied by swelling, lumpiness and a feeling of tightness which may be cyclical or non-cyclical in nature. Cyclical mastalgia is linked to the hormonal changes in the MENSTRUAL CYCLE but is more complex than was previously thought to be the case. Characteristically, symptoms are noticed in the days immediately before a period as a physical aspect of **PREMENSTRUAL SYNDROME**. In some women, breast symptoms can be apparent for as long as two weeks or from the time of ovulation until the onset of menstruation.

Most women probably experience mild symptoms of cyclical mastalgia at some stage in their reproductive life and the age range affected is broad, from the teenage years to the mid-forties. However, a significant number experience more acute and disabling symptoms which are severe enough to interfere with normal life.

It is now believed that sufferers from cyclical mastalgia are not only highly sensitive to normal, hormonal fluctuations, but that also, they are affected by certain dietary factors. In particular, it is thought that some women lack essential fatty acids that are found in evening primrose oil and fish oils, either because there is insufficient intake in their diet or due to inefficient utilisation by the body. Taking supplements has certainly been shown to help some sufferers although the improvement is not immediate but usually starts to be noticed after three or four months.

It is known that oestrogen is stored and released in small amounts by body fat hence cyclical mastalgia may be helped if an overweight woman reduces her weight. Also, a high intake of animal fat is believed to be another factor at work in cyclical mastalgia and reducing consumption may be helpful for some women and is also better for overall health.

However, it should be noted that dietary changes and the taking of supplements are not usually sufficient on their own to help women who suffer from severe cyclical mastalgia and medical treatment may need to be tried.

This takes the form of drug treatments, particularly danazol which is a powerful anti-hormonal preparation. This is often effective but it produces significant, unpleasant, side effects in about one quarter of the women for whom it is prescribed. Usually, if it is found to be helpful, the dose is reduced to the lowest level that has an effect as soon as possible. Even so, many doctors are unhappy about prescribing this potent drug for a prolonged period and may recommend that it is taken intermittently, perhaps only on certain days of the monthly cycle.

In the past, it was thought that the swelling, pain and lumpiness that is so much a feature of cyclical mastalgia was caused by fluid retention for which diuretics were prescribed. It is now known that fluid retention does not occur and so diuretic use is inappropriate.

Mastalgia can also be non-cyclical, i.e. occurring at any time and unrelated to the menstrual cycle. Frequently, a woman experiences a burning or stabbing pain, often only in one breast. Some of the conditions described above can be the cause but, not infrequently, the root of the problem lies elsewhere and pain is being referred to the breast. Muscular and skeletal problems (such as lung, digestive or heart problems, shingles and a condition called Tietze's syndrome which affects costal cartilage) can produce pain in the breast.

Non-cyclical mastalgia is a difficult condition to treat if no obvious cause is apparent but danazol may help some sufferers. Over-the-counter pain relief, relaxing in a hot bath and some 'alternative' remedies may help others, along with dietary changes, such as cutting down on the consumption of animal fat and ensuring that a good, balanced diet is being eaten.

INVERTED NIPPLES

Inverted nipples lie flat against the areola or are even turned inwards and appear to lie within a fold. This is due to the milk ducts being too short to allow the nipples to protrude and is only a problem if the woman wishes to breastfeed or is unhappy with her appearance.

The nipples can be encouraged to protrude by gentle manipulation or by wearing a suction device such as a nipple shield within the bra. Surgery to correct inverted nipples can be performed but it is usually not possible to breastfeed following this procedure.

BREAST CANCER

Breast cancer is the commonest cancer in women and is most common in post-menopausal women. The first signe of breast cancer that is usually noticed is a lump in the breast and/or a swollen lymph node in the armpit. In addition, there may be a change in the usual appearance of the breast or a puckering of skin in the region of the nipple. The breast may feel uncomfortable and there may be a discharge from the nipple. Most breast lumps are not serious but a woman who detects a lump should seek medical attention. (*See* **PREVENTATIVE MEASURES – PROTECTING THE BREASTS.**)

Treatment involves surgery, radiotherapy and chemotherapy and sometimes a combination of all three. Sometimes it is possible to remove a lump alone (a lumpectomy) but in other cases the whole breast has to be removed along with the lymph nodes under the arm. The degree of surgery depends on the size of the cancer and the extent to which it has spread.

The exact cause of breast cancer is unknown but some women are more at risk of developing the disease than others. There is a greater risk if a family member (especially a mother, aunt or sister) has had breast cancer or if the woman already has had benign breast tumours. Women who have not had children, those over the age of 30 at the birth of their first child, those who have not breastfed their babies and those who smoke are also at risk.

BREAST PLASTIC SURGERY

Breast plastic surgery consists of three types of plastic surgery performed on the breast; reduction, reconstruction and enlargement. The first two are almost always carried out for medical reasons whereas breast enlargement is usually cosmetic.

BREAST REDUCTION SURGERY

Breast reduction surgery is performed to decrease the size of very large breasts. It is the most straightforward of the three types of operation and it is performed both for physical and psychological reasons. The weight of large breasts causes strain on the neck, upper back and shoulders and women often develop poor posture as a result which can cause problems, particularly in later life. The skin between and beneath the breasts tends to get chafed, sweaty and sore and infection can easily occur. If the breasts are excessively large, feeding a baby is difficult, if not impossible, and many women give up as a result.

The psychological problems caused by large breasts can be immense and, inevitably, the woman finds herself receiving often unwelcome comments and attention from members of the opposite sex. All too often, assumptions are made by men about a female who is well-endowed and there is an unwillingness to acknowledge that there is a person with thoughts and feelings behind the breasts.

While some women may not mind about the attention they receive, for others, especially sensitive and self-conscious teenage girls, the situation can soon become intolerable. Typically, the young girl or woman habitually rounds her shoulders to try and hide her breasts or wears loose, baggy tops in an effort to conceal them. In the worst cases, she may be unwilling to attend school, go out with her friends or lead a normal life. Hence, although breast enlargement would not be considered appropriate for an unhappy teenager, reduction surgery for someone who is miserable would certainly be looked at sympathetically.

The waiting lists for, and availability of such operations on the National Health Service are, however, a source of problems. Breast reduction involves removing fat and other tissue to produce breasts of a smaller size but similar shape to the original. The nipple and areola have to be moved to a new position and this is most successful if each can be left attached to a stalk of breast tissue. If this is possible, then some nervous and blood supplies remain intact and there is a better chance of preserving sensitivity and the ability to breastfeed.

However, in some cases, the areola and nipple have to be cut off completely and then stitched into the new position as a graft. In this case, feeling and function are inevitably removed at least initially, and in fact, since the surgery may well result in cutting through milk ducts, most surgeons prefer women who may wish to breastfeed to wait until they have completed their family. Surgery inevitably produces scarring but the nature of this varies between individuals. Other possible complications include the development of residual, small, fatty lumps which usually disappear over time and the formation of an **ABSCESS** or ulcer in the vicinity of the wound.

BREAST RECONSTRUCTION SURGERY

The reason for breast reconstruction surgery is if a **MASTECTOMY** has been performed as part of cancer treatment. The timing of a reconstruction operation varies, with some specialists willing to perform the surgery immediately after removal of the cancerous breast. However, this is unlikely to be considered unless the surgeon is sure that the cancer has been caught at an early stage and that removal of part or all of the breast is the only treatment that is going to be required. Many specialists advise waiting to make sure that surgery has eliminated the cancer because if radiotherapy or chemotherapy were subsequently found to be necessary, they would adversely affect the success of reconstructive surgery.

A further point is that a woman who is initially horrified at the idea of losing a breast may find that she handles the reality of a mastectomy much better than she believed possible. As with any elective surgery, it is better to make a considered, reflective decision as to whether one wishes to proceed or not rather than rush in and regret one's haste at a later stage. For it is important to remember that although reconstructive surgery can build a substitute breast, it can never look or feel the same to the woman as the one which she has lost. A reconstructed breast removes the necessity of bothering to pad out a bra with a prosthesis and it will look normal beneath clothing. However, as with most surgery, there is a period of soreness and discomfort and potential disappointment may lie ahead for any woman who is not fully prepared. Having said this, the surgery may transform what has been a bad experience, with many women finding that their confidence is restored and that they then have the courage to get on with life after breast cancer.

The type of reconstructive surgery depends upon the extent of the original mastectomy. If sufficient breast tissue and skin are left, a silicone implant may suffice. Alternatively, a saline-filled implant may be used to expand the existing tissue before a permanent one in installed. The implants used are the same as those inserted for cosmetic surgery. Each consists of a silicone bag which is hemispherical in shape and filled either with gel or saline. Once in place, the implant behaves like normal tissue, i.e. it flattens when the woman lies down and feels natural when felt through the skin. Since there have been worrying health concerns attached to the use of earlier implants, considerable research has been directed towards producing types that are safe. However, safety remains a factor to be discussed by any woman considering having reconstructive surgery.

In some cases, where mastectomy has had to be radical and extensive, there is not enough skin or muscle left to support an implant. It then becomes necessary to take skin and muscle from the back or abdomen to use as a self-graft at the breast site, in order to eventually rebuild the breast with an implant. This is quite complicated surgery which can be painful during the recovery period and there is a risk of failure of the graft, which may fail to flourish in its new site.

A nipple can also be created, using skin from the inner thigh to produce an areola and tissue from the healthy nipple or an ear lobe to make the nipple itself. Once again, there is soreness initially while the surgical sites heal and for many women, who have already had extensive procedures, this is one operation too many, especially since it produces only an approximate result. Realistic-looking, synthetic nipples are available which simply stick on to the skin and many women prefer to use one of these or not to bother at all.

BREAST ENLARGEMENT SURGERY
Breast enlargement surgery is almost always regarded as cosmetic and is difficult, if not impossible, to obtain

on the NHS. This is in spite of the fact that for some women, the size of their breasts is a cause of considerable unhappiness and psychological distress. A few women have very little breast development at **PUBERTY** and this may be a source of great worry, even though it is considered to be normal for the individual concerned. The woman is often advised to wait until she has a baby because the surge of hormones, especially during a first pregnancy, can often cause the breasts to increase in size to quite a considerable extent.

However, a young woman may feel that this is rather a drastic solution compared to breast enlargement surgery, although it is important to bear in mind that implants have several implications as far as breastfeeding is concerned. Although breastfeeding is possible with implants in place, there is a natural risk of infections at this time. Infection can cause damage to the implant with the potential risk of rupture and leakage and the possible consequences of this (*see* below).

Also, there is considerable concern that slight, undetected leakages of gel or saline may be more common than previously suspected and may be passed on to the baby during breastfeeding, posing health risks for the child. For these reasons, many surgeons strongly advise young women who may want to breastfeed in the future, to delay having implants until they have completed their family. Also, breast enlargement for a girl in her teens who is still growing and developing, would not be considered by any reputable surgeon.

It is important for any woman considering breast enlargement to seriously examine her motives for doing so. Women seeking this procedure invariably believe that having larger breasts will make them more attractive. Hence they usually believe that they are less attractive as they are, whether this is, in fact, true or not as far as other people are concerned. If all goes well and the woman considers that the implants have been a success, she usually feels more attractive and self-confident.

However, the change stems from the way she now feels about herself and it is important to realize that people can build their self-confidence and self-esteem by means other than surgery. If the decision is made to proceed, it will be necessary to find a fairly substantial sum of money in order to pay for the operation at a private hospital. The procedure may also be available to women with private health care insurance as part of the overall package of benefits. It is essential to be realistic about what the final result of the surgery should be and to discuss all aspects of the procedure with the surgeon.

Small breasts cannot be made huge because, firstly, the change would be too drastic and, secondly, there may not be enough skin to stretch around the implants. The pressure on the natural breast tissue exerted by implants that are too large and taut may result in a distorted shape and a new set of problems. Most surgeons suggest a reasonable increase in size with the aim of producing the same shape of breast mound as before. Usually, the surgeon will have 'before' and 'after' photos of previous patients who have undergone the procedure. Hence a woman who is contemplating having the operation will be able to see for herself the type of changes that are made.

As mentioned above, the best time for a woman to have breast implants is after she has completed her family and finished breastfeeding. The basic procedure is to insert a pouch filled with sterile gel or saline either between the breast and pectoral muscles or under the muscles themselves. The operation requires a general anaesthetic but it is relatively straightforward and generally lasts for about one hour.

Post-operatively, there is inevitably a period of soreness, bruising and pain and the breasts have to be bandaged until healing is well underway. It is essential to wear a well-fitting support bra for the next few weeks and to watch out for signs of wound infection. Bruising and some degree of swelling may be present for up to six weeks. There is some scarring but the extent and site of this depends upon where the incision was made. It may be through and around the nipple, in the armpit or in the crease beneath the breast and will be about 5 cm in length.

There are a number of complications and health risks associated with the insertion of implants. Post-operatively, blood may continue to collect around the implant and this will necessitate removal of the implant and then reinsertion once the bleeding has stopped. If an infection occurs around or beneath the wound, the implant must once again be removed because of the danger of it becoming damaged. The infection will have to be treated and thoroughly cleared up with antibiotics, which may take some weeks, before the implant can be reinserted.

The most common problem is the formation of a hardened capsule, composed of fibrous scar tissue, which surrounds the implant so that it cannot move around. This can be intensely painful and can usually only be cured by cracking and breaking the scar tissue under general anaesthesia. Unfortunately, the capsule commonly re-forms and the woman may have to go through the process again or have the implants removed. It must be said that capsule formation was a greater problem with the earlier types of implants than it is with those used today but it still affects a propor-tion of women who undergo the procedure.

In the longer term, there is the risk of gel or saline leaking from the implant – a leakage which may go undetected but which can still have consequences for the health of the woman concerned. Particles of silicone gel from an implant have not only been discovered in nearby breast and lymph tissue but also in sites in the body that are much farther away. Numbers of women have suffered unpleasant symptoms and illnesses which they and some specialists believe are caused by an adverse reaction to silicone gel. In these instances, it may be that there is an autoimmune response set off by the presence of leaked particles which causes the body to attack its own tissues.

A number of court cases have been launched, particularly in North America, by women who are seeking compensation, claiming that their health has been ruined by implants. Some fatalities have also been blamed upon implants and there has been an increasing level of unease concerning their safety. A further area of concern is whether implants increase the risk of breast cancer, if only by making its detection more difficult, but there are conflicting views upon this.

If lumps of scar tissue or fatty deposits form as a result of disturbance caused by the operation, then these may raise alarm over the possibility of cancer being present. However, it is generally thought that the effectiveness of MAMMOGRAPHY is not reduced by the presence of implants. Many women undergo mammography before they have the implants inserted with repeat screening carried out at intervals afterwards, particularly if they experience problems.

It can be seen that there are many issues to be taken into account by those considering breast enlargement surgery but very many women continue to seek this procedure every year.

PREVENTATIVE MEASURES – PROTECTING THE BREASTS

The 'frontline' preventative measure for safeguarding the health of the breasts is SELF-EXAMINATION.

SELF-EXAMINATION

Self-examination should be carried out once a month, just before the onset of a period, in order to become fully familiar with the normal feel and appearance of the breasts so that any irregularities can be detected at an early stage and investigated, if necessary. It is recommended that women begin doing this by the age of 17 and continue the process beyond the MENOPAUSE and into older age. It is simple to perform and requires very little time. The procedure may be carried out as follows:

1 Stand in front of a mirror and become familiar with the normal appearance of the breast. Note skin texture and colour, whether both breasts are the same size or one is larger and whether one is positioned higher than the other. On a monthly basis, look for any alterations in appearance such as a slight change

in shape, a drawing in or retraction of a nipple, puckering or wrinkling of the skin or lightened or darkened colour and veins seeming more prominent than normal. Look for these changes with the arms held in different positions – loose by the side, hands on waist with elbows bent, raised above the head and hands placed on the head.

2 While in the bath or shower, use the fingers of the opposite hand to become familiar with how each breast feels to the touch. The slight lumpiness is quite normal and is due to the natural composition of the breast tissue. Every month, methodically check each breast, working round in a clockwise fashion. Feel for any unusual lump, thickening or tenderness, remembering that these can occur quite normally, especially before a period. Raise the arm behind the head and check the breast again and also the armpit looking for any enlargement or tenderness in the lymph nodes. Feel the nipple and squeeze it gently, looking for any unusual discharge or bleeding.

3 If a lump or other irregularity is detected, have it checked by your GP who will, if necessary, arrange for a consultation with a specialist for further investigation. Try not to worry, even if this does take place, since most breast lumps are benign and those that are not are usually treatable.

Mammography is a screening technique involving X-ray examination of the breast, resulting in an image on film called a mammogram. It is used to detect potentially malignant spots of breast tissue at an early stage and is one of the techniques employed in the diagnosis of cancer. Ultrasound scanning and thermography are other diagnostic techniques that are particularly useful in women aged under 50 in whom breast tissue is too dense to obtain clear results with mammography.

Mammography involves compressing each breast between two plates enclosed within a machine, in front of which the woman stands. Up to three images of each breast are usually obtained on the first screening. The process, which is very quick, lasting only a few minutes, causes discomfort but is not painful and all women aged between 50 and 64 years in the UK are invited for screening every three years. It is possible that the age range may change in the future, with both older and younger women being offered mammography if it is felt to be beneficial. If malignancy is present, it is revealed as a dense white patch on the mammogram at a stage before it can be felt by manual examination. Prompt detection of breast cancer offers the hope of less radical and invasive treatment and a greater chance of an early and complete cure.

Thermography is a method of recording the heat produced in different areas of the body using photographic film sensitive to infrared radiation. Areas with a copious blood circulation generate more heat and this situation occurs abnormally if a tumour is present. The film image produced is called a thermogram and the technique is regarded as particularly valuable in the detection of breast cancer.

CHAPTER 7

Sexual fulfilment and enjoyment

The person who could devise one simple formula to enable all people to achieve a fulfilled and enjoyable sex life would be rich and famous indeed! Since sex has emerged from the shadows as a subject that can be openly discussed, few areas of human experience have attracted such a sustained level of universal interest. However, in spite of all the volumes that have been written on this subject and the many hours that have been devoted to its discussion, the achievement of sexual fulfilment remains elusive for many people. This is because every individual is different and so each person's experience of sex is unique and personal.

People do not start off from the same baseline, or even need to reach the same level of enjoyment in their sexual lives, for some to feel fulfilled and others dissatisfied. It is generally believed that men have a greater need for sex than women but that they are more readily satisfied because the attainment of orgasm is felt to be easier for them. Whether this is true or not, it may be of little comfort to the individual man who feels that something in his sex life is lacking, even if he is able to achieve orgasm. Also, there are enormous differences between individuals of the same gender, producing men and women with greater, lesser and similar levels of sexual desire and aspiration who may or may not be compatible in their relationships. Although this is a highly complex area of human experience, it is possible for some general observations to be made.

Probably the most well-known factor, and one which most people eventually discover for themselves, is that sexual fulfilment is achieved not only through the body but also through the mind. Perhaps for many people, especially those who are young, the physical aspects of sex seem sufficient, at least for a time. However, for many others and possibly more particularly for women, this is not enough and they find that sexual fulfilment cannot be achieved unless feelings and emotions are fully engaged.

SEXUAL AROUSAL AND RESPONSE

The physical aspects of sexual fulfilment, which are usually equated with the achievement of orgasm, are essentially similar for both men and women with the same physiological responses occurring in both sexes. Physiological responses take two forms; vasocongestion, in which there is an increased flow of blood into erectile tissue so that it enlarges and stiffens and myotonia, in which muscles contract. Sexual arousal and response have been divided into four phases: excitement, plateau, orgasm and resolution.

These take place as an increasing and then declining continuum of sexual response with orgasm or climax as the definitive moment. In practice, the first two phases may be difficult to distinguish from one another and in men, they are marked by enlargement and erection of the penis and an increase in size of the testicles. Additionally, muscles in the lower abdominal region may contract. In women, there is similar enlargement of the clitoris, breasts and labia and release of lubricating vaginal secretions. The inner portion of the vagina expands and lengthens slightly while the outer part becomes congested and the uterus becomes lifted from the pelvic floor. The vaginal walls deepen in colour and a reddening flush may spread across the abdomen, breasts and neck. The changes in the uterus and vagina create a depression in which sperm may be received. Muscles in the lower abdomen or elsewhere in the body may contract and in both men and women, heartbeat and breathing rate increases. Women usually require more direct physical stimulation from their partner, for a longer period of time, to reach a peak of sexual arousal than is the case for men. However, for both men and women, sexual foreplay can be intensely pleasurable with the partner's increasing level of arousal intensifying their own response.

Orgasm in both sexes involves rhythmic contractions within the reproductive organs, culminating in an intensely pleasurable climactic release. In men, this process involves firstly the release of semen into the urethra by the various glands involved (emission). The second stage is ejaculation, in which one final reflex contraction of the urethra, reproductive organs and muscles forcibly ejects the semen from the urethral opening. In women, the outer portion of the vagina contracts rhythmically but the inner two thirds do not. The uterus and muscles of the pelvic floor and lower abdomen also contract, culminating in a final, pleasurable release of tension. However, women may also experience more than one orgasm which may vary in intensity. In both sexes, the orgasm stage is brief, occupying just a few seconds. During the final, resolution stage, the reproductive organs gradually reassume their pre-arousal size and heartbeat rate and breathing return to normal. There follows a refractory period, which varies in length, in which it is difficult for the person to become sexually aroused again.

MASTURBATION, SEXUAL FANTASY AND ROLE PLAY

Although masturbation, sexual fantasy and role play are common and normal, they remain, even in this sexually enlightened age, slightly 'taboo' and a cause of unease for many people. Masturbation is physical self-stimulation of the external genital organs in order to produce sexual pleasure and possibly orgasm. It is considered to be a normal part of childhood and adolescence and is carried out by many adults as well, although they would not necessarily admit to this being the case. Masturbation may be carried out both by those within and outside of a fulfilling sexual relationship.

Unfortunately, many people carry about an unnecessary burden of guilt with regard to masturbation. It is normal, not harmful in any way and can be highly therapeutic and helpful for those who feel inhibited about their body or sexuality. A person who enjoys masturbation is neither more or less sexually complete than anybody else and problems only arise when the person, or his or her partner, feel in some way threatened by the activity.

Much of the above also applies to sexual fantasies which are equally indulged in by men and women but are often kept a secret even from a loved and trusted partner. People may feel guilty about their fantasies, particularly because they often involve someone other than their partner. Or, they may feel guilty about the content of their fantasy and worry that they may be somehow abnormal for needing to indulge in it in the first place.

It is important to remember that fantasies involve make-believe scenarios in which the person would usually not involve him or herself in real life. Usually a subject of private thought, they are commonplace and are only harmful if the person having them allows him or herself to become beset with guilt. However, some people like to go a little farther and act out their fantasies in role play, often with a trusted partner, and as long as both are happy and willing to take part, then there is no harm in this either.

PROBLEMS OF SEXUAL PERFORMANCE AND ENJOYMENT AND THEIR TREATMENT

The experience of sexual response and orgasm is a highly individual one which often varies from one occasion to another. Women may have difficulty in reaching orgasm at all, but sexual problems are frequent in people of both sexes (*see* below). Also, it is quite common for people to feel vaguely dissatisfied or that their experiences do not measure up to some ideal that they may or may not have achieved before. In this context, it is probably true to say that people now have higher expectations than in the past through being exposed to so much information about sex in the media and in broadcasting. As stated previously, an enormous number of psychological, emotional and other factors in life can and do affect a person's enjoyment of sex and these are referred to in greater detail in this section.

It is certain that almost all people experience dissatisfaction in their sexual life at some stage or other. For many, the situation may be a temporary one, relating to a difficulty in a relationship or other aspect of life which can be worked through and resolved. Others may not be particularly concerned, preferring to concentrate on other areas of their life from which they can gain fulfilment. For some, however, difficulties become severe enough to make them seek professional help and it is important to emphasize that sexual problems can very often be resolved in this way. If the person is involved in a long-term relationship, it is quite possible that both partners may need to co-operate in a treatment programme, even if it is apparently only one of them who is affected. Some of the more common problems of sexual performance are discussed below.

REDUCTION IN SEXUAL DESIRE (LIBIDO)

A reduction in libido is universally experienced by both men and women at some stage in their life, even if it is only transitory and occurring at times of physical illness. Almost any disease, illness or physical injury can cause a lowering of libido, as can the drugs used in their treatment, or any drug or alcohol abuse. If an illness is likely to be short-lived, then the problem will probably be readily accepted as one which will resolve itself once the person has recovered physically. If it is more severe or long-lasting, then it may still be possible to help, perhaps through an adjustment in medication or psychosexual therapy. It may be the psychological impact of the condition that is causing the loss of libido. For example, if a person has been disfigured as a result of an accident or cancer treatment, such as **MASTECTOMY**, the person's self-confidence may need to be built up again through counselling which involves the loving support of the partner, when appropriate.

Psychological causes for a lowered libido are numerous, ranging from illnesses, such as depression, to stress, which can itself have many different sources. Work, family and financial worries can cause enormous degrees of stress and exhaustion and, all too often, the libido is one of the first casualties, thereby compounding the problems that already exist. Women commonly experience a reduced desire for sex after the birth of a baby and this is due to a combination of hormonal changes and tiredness caused by the demands of looking after the new arrival.

All sorts of anxieties and insecurities within a relationship can also caused a lowered libido. A person may worry about the extent or nature of the emotional attachment felt by the partner or doubt his or her own sexual attractiveness and ability to please. Such anxieties, whether conscious or subconscious, can all ultimately result in a lessening of desire, as can thoughts and feelings which are acknowledged but unexpressed. In long-term relationships especially, boredom can all too easily creep in. People obviously become used to each other and may find it harder to sustain the excitement that they felt at the start of their relationship.

It is extremely important for couples to make time for each other and to work hard at their sexual relationship, perhaps discovering new aspects of lovemaking, so that they continue to find fulfilment and enjoyment in this important part of their life. Other relevant factors are previously traumatic sexual encounters, especially **RAPE** which, not surprisingly, leaves people psychologically scarred and makes the resumption of any kind of a sexual life extremely difficult.

Resolving a loss of, or lowered, libido, obviously depends upon the cause of the problem. As mentioned above, truly physical causes resulting directly from some medical condition may well be amenable to treatment or counselling which can bring about an improvement. Psychological reasons require that the cause be identified and removed, or at least lessened. The most important way of bringing this about is to be prepared to openly and honestly discuss the problem. Since it usually arises within a relationship, the best course of action is to talk it through with the partner but many people find this very difficult. A sex therapist or counsellor can help a couple to discuss matters in a non-judgemental way and suggest practical ways in which problems can be overcome.

MALE PROBLEMS

Apart from the loss of libido discussed above, men commonly experience one or two other difficulties in sexual performance at some stage in life. Often these are transient in nature but nevertheless, they can be a cause of anxiety and stress, undermining self-esteem and placing a strain on any relationship in which a man is involved. Also, it is true to say that something which may be regarded as just a difficulty for one man may become a problem for another.

As with so many aspects of sexual health, embarrassment often prevents a man from seeking professional help and he may even find it difficult to confide in his partner. It is certainly far more beneficial to discuss a problem openly than to pretend that nothing is wrong. Talking things over with his partner and seeking help from his GP, in the first instance, enables the man to take the initiative and this, in itself, may help to resolve the problem. A GP may well investigate aspects of physical health and enquire about lifestyle factors such as levels of stress to see if there is any apparent cause. If necessary, the man (and his partner) may be referred for specialist help in the form of psychosexual therapy and counselling.

Impotence

Impotence is usually defined as the inability to have sexual intercourse due to failure to achieve or maintain an erection. It also describes the situation in which an erection is achieved but there is a failure to achieve orgasm and ejaculation. There are a range of causes including certain diseases or conditions such as diabetes mellitus and some hormonal disorders. Also, alcohol or drug abuse, smoking and obesity may contribute to the problem, which can additionally arise as a side effect of taking some prescription drugs.

In the elderly, some cases of impotence are caused by low levels of testosterone and this can be corrected by **HORMONE REPLACEMENT THERAPY.** Also, men in older age often find that they require more prolonged stimulation in order to achieve an erection than was the case when they were younger, but this is regarded as a factor of ageing rather than impotence. Most commonly, the cause of impotence is psychogenic, resulting from stress, anxiety, grief or other emotional trauma which may be (but is often not) related to any particular relationship in which the man is involved. Impotence, in itself, causes further stress and a loss of self-esteem and this further perpetuates the problem and is likely to place great strain on a relationship, even when a partner is loving and supportive.

Treatment for impotence depends upon the cause. If organic, i.e. relating to a medical condition, physical state or lifestyle, then measures such as altering medication, pelvic floor exercises to improve muscle tone, losing weight, giving up smoking and reducing alcohol consumption, may be recommended. Also, there are a variety of specialized devices such as particular forms of condom and a pump which can help to produce an erection.

Various drugs are also available and the one which has caused intense recent interest is Viagra™ which is medically known as sildenafil. This drug acts to block or slow down the action of an enzyme called phospodiesterase, which is one of the agents responsible for the loss of penile erection. If the drug is taken before sexual intercourse, it acts to maintain an erection when the penis is stimulated by delaying the operation of the enzyme.

Although hailed as a 'wonder drug' and one which generated an almost frenzied demand amongst men with impotence problems, Viagra™ is not suitable for everyone. It is contra-indicated and could be harmful if taken by men suffering from a variety of illnesses and medical conditions. It also produces a range of possible side-effects, some of which are unpleasant. Hence any man considering taking Viagra™ needs to be fully informed about the effects of the drug and will require a physical check-up and discussion with his doctor. The drug is expensive and although it can now be more freely prescribed than when it was first introduced, it is still not necessarily available to all.

If the cause of the impotence is psychogenic, then talking about the problem and taking steps to, for example, alleviate stress or remove the source of worry is the best possible treatment. It may be feasible to accomplish this without professional help, depending upon the cause of the anxiety. Professional help, if needed, may take the form of counselling to suggest means of avoiding stress, perhaps by making lifestyle changes and possibly, short-term use of antidepressants. If anxiety can be relieved, then the problem of impotence will often be resolved as well.

If necessary, a referral can be made for sexual therapy and counselling which is particularly helpful for those in committed relationships who are prepared to work together to overcome the problem.

Premature ejaculation
Premature ejaculation, in which orgasm habitually occurs too soon to be satisfying for either partner, is the most commonly reported male sexual problem. It affects nearly all men at some stage in life and particularly those in younger age groups. Anxiety about previous experiences of premature ejaculation greatly increases the chances of it happening again and undermines self-esteem.

Resuming lovemaking after one episode of premature ejaculation usually helps, but a squeeze technique can also be employed which is simple to carry out and effective. It may be carried out either by the man himself or his partner and involves squeezing the end of the penis to delay impending ejaculation, even if only for a few moments. With practice, control over the timing of ejaculation can usually be achieved so that orgasm then takes place at a point which is more satisfactory to both partners.

Failure to achieve orgasm

Failure to achieve orgasm has usually been regarded as a female problem but it is one which frequently affects men also. In men, it describes the situation in which initial sexual arousal produces an erection, but this is lost before climax is reached.

The cause may be physical, with excess consumption of alcohol or exhaustion on a particular occasion being the most common reason. In this case, the problem is only likely to be transient in nature. If it is more persistent, then there is almost certainly a psychological reason behind the problem, the nature of which may or may not be apparent.

There may be an emotional problem connected to the relationship with the partner, particularly if the man has been deeply hurt before. Also, experience of previous sexual abuse can make entering into a sexual relationship extremely difficult and lead to problems of this kind.

Sexual therapy, particularly when undertaken with the help of an understanding partner, will usually resolve this problem in due course.

FEMALE PROBLEMS

In common with men, women may experience several problems which prevent them from having an enjoyable and fulfilling sexual life. Some of these may have an identifiable, physical cause but very often, the problem is a possibly unacknowledged, psychological or emotional one. In Western society, in which sex and the enjoyment of sex pervades the media, a woman who experiences problems can very easily feel inadequate.

This is particularly the case since women are apt to blame themselves if they do not scale the heights of sexual performance. They all too easily feel guilty if, for example, they do not reach orgasm in response to their partner's lovemaking. Many conceal the true state of things or pretend to responses that they do not feel for fear of hurting their partner's feelings, or worry about the consequences for the relationship that revelation may bring. Depression, strained or broken relationships and avoidance of sex can all too often result if no attempt is made to resolve problems. Talking about problems, with the partner and/or with an appropriate professional, is the first step in achieving a solution.

Failure of orgasm

When sex is portrayed in films or on television programmes, it nearly always portrays the woman reaching orgasm simultaneously with her partner in a passionate and often noisy encounter! This is very much depicted as being the normal experience which everyone should expect all of the time. However, the reality is somewhat different for many women for at least some of the time. Some women have never had an orgasm while for others, it happens only rarely.

The reasons for this are almost never physical (unless the woman is unfortunate enough to have been subjected to CIRCUMCISION), but are commonly attributable to lack of stimulation and poor technique or to psychological problems.

Nearly all women require physical stimulation, usually of the clitoris, to become sexually aroused initially and this may need to be continued in order for them to reach orgasm. Intercourse itself may simply not be enough and in these circumstances, the woman and her partner need to discover what is right for her. This may need to be a process of self-discovery through MASTURBATION and some women can only reach orgasm if they masturbate during sex. Also, and hardly surprisingly, a woman is not likely to have an orgasm if a sexual encounter is, for any reason, causing her discomfort or pain.

A whole range of psychological and emotional problems can prevent a woman from experiencing orgasm, either on a particular occasion or on a more consistent basis. These include feelings of insecurity within a relationship, unresolved guilt or fears about sex itself (stemming perhaps from previous bad experiences), stress and worry in other areas of life, lack of confidence about sexual attractiveness and unwillingness to communicate sexual needs. A woman may also be unwilling to give herself completely during lovemaking, perhaps because she is afraid of losing self-control or of the implications which intimacy might bring. It is known that almost any psychological or emotional difficulty may affect a woman's ability to enjoy sex and experience orgasm. However, these problems can, in the great majority of cases, be overcome. Therapy can help to identify the nature of the problem, which is particularly useful when this is not apparent to the woman herself, and methods of overcoming it can then be devised.

Vaginismus

Vaginismus is a sudden and involuntary contraction of the muscles surrounding the vaginal opening, very often involving other abdominal muscles as well as those of the buttocks and thighs, which occurs during lovemaking and prevents penetration. Women of any age can be affected and most believe that the spasm of the muscles occurs as a result of a physical disorder. In fact, the response occurs because the woman subconsciously wishes to prevent penetrative sex for reasons which she may not be aware of herself. The condition can affect young and sexually inexperienced women but it can also arise in those who were previously able to allow intimate contact. Affected women may be able to enjoy intimacy which does not involve penetrative sex and the condition may not be a problem for them. Others, however, worry to such an extent that they may avoid developing intimate relationships out of fear and embarrassment.

There may be some obvious reason for vaginismus such as a previous traumatic or painful experience of sex. However, more subtle psychological factors may equally be at work, for example, guilt or feelings that sex is somehow shameful, dirty or undesirable. A mother's distaste for sex can easily be passed on to a daughter creating problems for the child when she grows up.

Young, inexperienced women may simply be fearful due to ignorance about sexual and reproductive function and about their own bodies. Women who suffer from vaginismus can usually be taught to overcome the problem if they seek professional help, which may involve both physical and psychological therapy.

Physical therapy involves teaching the woman to use vaginal dilators which are made of rubber or glass and are cylindrical in shape and of different diameters. The woman starts off with the narrowest one and learns to gently insert and remove this herself before moving up to the next size. Eventually, she may be encouraged to allow her partner to insert the dilators so that she is gradually able to overcome her fear. Alternatively, a couple may be counselled to enjoy other types of lovemaking which do not involve penetration until the woman is able to relax and feel confident about having full sexual relations.

Psychological therapy seeks to discover and overcome deeper fears about sex through discussion and counselling. A combination of methods over a period of time helps most women to overcome vaginismus.

Frigidity

Frigidity describes a complete lack of desire for sex and often, the person feels revulsion at the idea of sex and may dislike being touched. Psychological factors are a common cause of frigidity, and, in particular, ideas that were acquired in childhood such as the belief that sex is dirty (or shameful or sinful). The person concerned may have been brought up by parents who were emotionally removed and did not demonstrate love for the child or for each other.

Additionally, frigidity may stem from an earlier traumatic sexual experience such as abuse in childhood or rape. This is especially likely if the experience has been suppressed and not acknowledged. Psychosexual therapy can usually help a woman to gradually explore and overcome the problems that are the cause of frigidity but the process may take some time.

Painful sexual intercourse or dyspareunia

Painful sexual intercourse can have numerous causes, many of which are physical but some are psychological. The pain itself may be localized (i.e. confined to the vaginal/genital region) or arise from deeper within the pelvis and lower abdomen. Vaginal and genital pain may be caused by infections such as THRUSH, TRICHOMONAS and GENITAL HERPES (*see* SEXUALLY TRANS-MITTED DISEASES).

Vaginal dryness due to a lack of foreplay and sexual arousal can result in pain during intercourse and this may also be a problem during and after the MENOPAUSE due to a loss of hormones. Allergic reactions or irritation within the vagina may be caused by spermicidal preparations or the rubber of a CONDOM or DIAPHRAGM, resulting in localized pain during intercourse. Bruising in the genital region or an episiotomy or perineal scar after childbirth are further causes.

Deeper pelvic pain during intercourse may result from PELVIC INFLAMMATORY DISEASE (PID), FIBROIDS, ENDOMETRIOSIS, ABDOMINAL ADHESIONS following surgery or cancer treatment, PROLAPSED UTERUS or VAGINAL and URINARY TRACT INFECTIONS. Psychological causes are similar to those underlying a **LOSS OF LIBIDO** and **FRIGIDITY** which have been described above. A psychological problem can very easily be translated into a real physical pain which is felt during intercourse but for which there is no discernible organic cause. Treatment for dyspareunia obviously depends upon the cause and a woman who consistently experiences painful intercourse should always seek medical advice.

Female genital mutilation

Sometimes referred to as female circumcision, female genital mutilation refers to the practice of removing the clitoris and sometimes the labia of young girls and sewing together the remaining tissue, just leaving a small opening to allow for the passage of urine and menstrual blood. The procedure is carried out for cultural and religious reasons in many parts of Africa and although it is usually officially banned, the practice is difficult to stamp out.

Female circumcision is never justified on medical grounds. It is often performed in unhygienic conditions and deaths from infection and septicaemia are not unusual. Urinary tract and pelvic infections are common later because the flow of urine and menstrual blood may be impeded. Sexual intercourse can be extremely difficult for women who have undergone genital mutilation and they are often left unable to enjoy sex. Corrective surgery can improve the situation with regard to urination and menstruation and lessen the risks of pelvic infections. A woman who is suffering as a result of genital mutilation carried out in childhood should seek medical advice.

CHAPTER 8

Rape

It is beyond the scope of this book to discuss this horrendous crime in any detail, beyond stating those aspects which have become fairly common knowledge. It is certain that an enormous number of rapes go unreported and that women (and men) of any age can be victims. It is the case that male rape is being increasingly reported and that male victims suffer a great deal and sometimes in an additional way because rape crisis centres and services tend to be geared towards the needs of women.

Most rapes are carried out by assailants who are known to their victims and the association varies from slight acquaintances to friends and family members. Due to this, many victims torture themselves with feelings of guilt and worry that they may have somehow given unknowing encouragement to their assailant. It is a mistake to feel this way. Pleas made by a rapist in court that he was 'led on' by his victim are simply excuses made to try and justify his criminal behaviour. This is because rape has more to do with the

exercise of abusive power than it has with sexual grati-
fication and hence non-consent is an essential trigger
for the rapist.

Unfortunately, it is not outwardly obvious that
someone is prepared to abuse power in this way, nor are
the circumstances necessarily apparent. Many rapists
appear to have previously led ordinary sorts of lives and
it is only sometimes that particular traits of character or
past history provides clues for their behaviour.

Rape would be severe enough if it ended with the
complete sexual and physical violation that is
involved, often with the accompaniment of extreme
fear. However, it usually leaves psychological and
emotional scars that last well beyond the act itself
which can ruin the victim's future life. In the
immediate aftermath, a huge range of emotions can be
experienced which commonly include feelings of
degradation and disgust, extreme anger, guilt, shame,
fear and shock to the extent of numbness and
withdrawal. Many victims feel an overwhelming need
to take a bath or shower and to throw away or destroy
clothing that was worn during the attack. If the rape is
to be reported to the police with a view to pressing
charges, it is important that none of this takes place.

Unfortunately, the victim needs to be examined by a
police doctor and her clothing retained to provide
forensic evidence. All police forces now have highly
trained and sympathetic officers to deal with rape

victims and they will provide all necessary support and help in the aftermath of an attack. The victims is treated with respect and understanding and helped through the ordeal of making a statement and undergoing a medical examination. Seeing a doctor is additionally important as there may be a need for the victim to receive advice on preventing or treating any sexually transmitted infection and for the provision of **EMERGENCY CONTRA-CEPTION**. The victim may well be in no fit state to think of these matters at the time but it is important that they are dealt with as soon as possible.

Many victims do not feel up to facing the ordeal of going to the police and reporting the crime. Rape crisis centres exist to provide sympathetic and professional help and counselling for victims and continuing support. The Samaritans also provide a similar support service over the anonymity of the telephone. In the longer term, it is usually essential for healing that the rape and the feelings that it has engendered are freely discussed with someone whom the victim trusts. Professional counsellors can help, as can family and friends, but the healing process may be a long and painful one. Future sexual relationships are one obvious area of difficulty and marriages and partner-ships may or may not be strengthened or destroyed under the strain. A great deal depends upon the nature not only of the victim but also of those with whom she or he is involved but talking will help rather than harm.

CHAPTER 9

Sexual development
and puberty

The differentiation of both external and internal sexual
and reproductive organs and structures begins at about
the 8th week of foetal development. Differentiation
itself depends upon whether the embryo is male and
possesses XY sex chromosomes or female with XX sex
chromosomes. The sex chromosomes ultimately determine whether male or female hormones will be
released, under the influence of which the reproductive
organs begin to develop. Prior to the 8th week of
pregnancy, the appearance of the external genital region
is the same in both male and female foetuses. The
genitalia develop from a primordial structure called the
genital tubercle while the internal organs begin to form
under the influence of circulating hormones.

By the time of birth, the sexual and reproductive
organs and structures are fully formed and contain
their complement of sex cells, as described previously
(*see* **STRUCTURE AND FUNCTION OF THE REPRODUCTIVE**

ORGANS). In both boys and girls, two sets of changes occur at puberty: the reproductive organs become fully mature and functional, and the child acquires the secondary sexual characteristics which are the defining features of adulthood.

PUBERTY IN BOYS

Puberty is the period of physical development during which a boy attains sexual maturity. The average age of onset is between 12 and 14 years but it may be earlier or later depending upon individual genetic factors. The changes at puberty are brought about by the release of hormones with the process being initiated by the pituitary gland at the base of the brain.

The gland secretes gonadotrophins (gonadotrophic hormones) in the form of follicle stimulating hormones (FSH) and interstitial cell stimulating hormones (ICSH) which are carried by the bloodstream to the testicles. Here, FSH stimulates the growth and maturation of sperm while ICSH is responsible for the production and release of androgens, especially testosterone, by the interstitial cells (*see* **STRUCTURE AND FUNCTION OF THE MALE REPRODUCTIVE ORGANS**).

Under the influence of testosterone, a series of gradual but dramatic changes occur which follow a particular sequence:

1 Enlargement of the scrotum and testicles
2 Elongation and enlargement of the penis

3 Growth of pubic hair followed by underarm, body and facial hair

In addition, there is a spurt of muscular and skeletal growth with the boy more or less reaching his adult height and weight by the end of puberty. A further change involves the gradual enlargement of the vocal cords so that the voice 'breaks' and deepens to that of an adult man. The 'Adam's apple' which is a projection of the thyroid cartilage of the larynx becomes more visible and prominent as the boy matures.

Mature sperm are being produced by around the age of 14 to 16, depending upon the timing of the onset of puberty. However, maximum male fertility is not attained until the late teens and twenties.

The surge in hormones is frequently associated with a particular scourge of puberty, the development of acne. Teenage acne occurs because the sebaceous glands in the skin become more active under hormonal influence and secrete more sebum (an oily substance) leading to blockage, infection and the development of pustules. This common condition can be a source of misery for a teenage boy, occurring at a time when he is likely to be particularly self-conscious about his appearance. Once hormone levels have reached equilibrium at the end of puberty, acne usually disappears. However, it must be taken seriously by parents and others, handled sensitively and never made the subject of jokes or teasing. If it is particularly severe, the family doctor should be consulted as both prescription and over-the-counter preparations can help as can a vigilant skin cleansing routine.

Hormonal imbalance during puberty may also result in a slight and temporary enlargement of the breasts of a boy (since the testicles also secrete small amounts of the female hormone, oestrogen). This can also cause serious alarm and embarrassment for a boy, who may well need to receive reassurance from the family doctor that he is not abnormal and all is well.

Finally, for most boys, puberty sees the start of the occasional occurrence of 'wet dreams' or ejaculation during night-time sleep. Once again, this may be personally embarrassing for a boy but he will have hopefully been told that this is a universal, normal experience and so it will not become a cause of anxiety.

PUBERTY IN GIRLS

The onset of puberty in girls usually occurs between the ages of 10 to 14 but may be earlier (precocious puberty)or later, depending upon individual genetic factors. Puberty lasts for about five years and, as in boys, is initiated by the release of hormones from the pituitary gland which then act directly upon the sexual organs. The most dramatic event for girls is the onset of MENSTRUATION (menarche) in response to the production and release of the female hormones, oestrogen and progesterone. The ovaries mature and begin to release eggs and the uterus enlarges, along with development and maturation of the genital organs. A period of accelerated growth with a gain in height and weight accompanies these changes. The hips broaden and the pattern of fat distribution changes to produce the characteristic female body shape. Also, the secondary sexual characteristics develop as puberty progresses, most notably the enlargement of the breasts, growth of pubic and underarm hair and the development of sweat glands.

By the end of puberty, a girl has attained most of her adult height and weight although growth and maturation continue until about the age of 18. In girls, growth, breast development and the appearance of hair usually precede menarche, which is dependent upon the attainment of a certain critical weight. This is the proportion of body fat compared to lean tissue which seems to be required before menarche is reached and regular menstrual periods are maintained. During the years of puberty, the ratio of lean to fat tissue changes from 5:1 to 3:1 at menarche. This represents an increase in fat tissue of 125 per cent over a period of two to three years – fat which produces a small amount of oestrogen. This helps to explain why plump girls often begin to menstruate at an earlier age than thin ones. The exact role of fatty tissue in stimulating the production of female hormones remains unclear.

However, women who lose weight due to eating disorders or through high levels of physical activity (such as athletes and ballerinas), often have very irregular periods or fail to menstruate at all (amenorrhoea). Normal menstrual cycles are usually resumed once weight is regained.

It is obviously important that girls are well-prepared beforehand for the physical changes that they will go through at puberty and that menstruation, in particular, is thoroughly explained.

CHAPTER 10

Contraception

Prevention of pregnancy was formerly regarded as a problem mainly for women, but attitudes have slowly been changing, although there is still a long way to go with regard to the education of young people (*see* Chapter 12). One encouraging, recent development has been the advent of a male hormonal pill, which has increased the range of contraceptive options open to men and has been generally welcomed, especially by those in committed relationships.

The need to prevent unplanned pregnancy and to educate young people about contraception and make it freely available to them are controversial subjects that have become firmly fixed on the political agenda. This has been brought about because of the unpalatable fact that Britain has the highest rate of teenage pregnancy of any country in Europe. Of equal concern is the huge rise in the incidence of **SEXUALLY TRANSMITTED DISEASES** which have increased by 50 per cent in recent years, particularly among teenagers and young people. Some of the barrier methods of contraception have, of course, an enormously important role to play in the prevention of these infections and this aspect, which has been dubbed 'safe sex', is discussed at the end of this chapter.

Contraception literally means 'against conception' and there are a number of different methods available which work to prevent pregnancy in two main ways. The majority act by making it difficult for sperm and egg to meet while a minority make it unlikely that any fertilized egg will be able to implant in the womb. Some of the more recent advanced methods employ a combination of both these strategies in order to prevent pregnancy.

CONTRACEPTIVE METHODS

NATURAL FAMILY PLANNING

Natural family planning does not involve the use of any artificial barrier or chemical device but is based on calculating a woman's fertile period and abstaining from sex during this time. The fertile period lasts from seven days before OVULATION until one day after it, i.e. a minimum time of eight days. This is based on the fact that sperm can survive for up to one week within the female reproductive system and an ovulated egg is viable for 24 hours.

Obviously, for natural family planning to be successful, the time of ovulation must be able to be accurately calculated and since there is considerable room for error, couples using this method may wish to abstain for sex for longer than eight days in order to avoid pregnancy.

The predicted time of ovulation is usually calculated by a combination of different methods. This involves ongoing recording of the timing of menstruation for at least six months. Ovulation usually occurs 14 days before a monthly period and so a pattern can usually be detected during the recording process. Also, the woman takes her resting temperature each morning when she wakes up, with the norm being 37° C. The temperature usually drops slightly just prior to ovulation but then rises by 0.2° C when this occurs. It then remains elevated until the onset of menstruation.

Changes take place in the quantity and consistency of the cervical mucus during the menstrual cycle and so this is checked by the woman on a daily basis. As ovulation approaches, the mucus becomes clearer, more slippery and often more profuse. But after the egg is released it become sticky, thick and whitish and generally more inhospitable to sperm. Some women experience a slight pain, low down on the same side as the ovary that is releasing the egg at ovulation. Also, the breasts may be tender or there may be a slight discharge of blood to indicate that ovulation is taking place. Changes also occur in the cervix itself throughout the menstrual cycle, under hormonal influence, which can be detected with practice.

However, all these indicators, which are usually grouped under the heading of the sympto-thermic method of natural birth control, can be difficult to ascertain and are subject to variation.

It can be seen that to practise natural birth control requires determination and commitment, patience and self-control in both the woman and her partner. The method can work very well for a couple in a stable, long-term relationship where both partners are prepared to accept the restraints that following it imposes. Calculating the timing of ovulation is also useful for those **PLANNING CONCEPTION** and one of the further advantages of sympto-thermic methods is that a woman becomes intimately familiar with the natural workings of her own body.

There are commercially available methods of measuring a woman's hormone levels for contraceptive purposes, such as the Persona™ method, which have come about because of the need to find out when a woman is most fertile and therefore most likely to conceive.

Such a method consists of a small hand-held computerised monitor and test sticks which collect hormones from early morning urine and convert them into a form that can be read by the monitor. The monitor gets to know a woman's monthly cycle and displays a green light when the woman can safely have sexual intercourse without using contraceptives and a red light when she is at risk of getting pregnant. Typically it will identify 6 to 10 'red' days. This method has the advantage of being completely natural but it does not offer protection against **SEXUALLY TRANSMITTED DISEASES**.

CERVICAL CAP

A cervical cap is a cap-shaped rubber device, more or less circular in shape, which is a barrier method of contraception designed to physically prevent sperm from reaching an egg. There are three slightly different designs and each comes in a number of different sizes. The correct size needs to be determined by a doctor and instruction given to the woman so that she can learn to fit the device correctly. The cap is inserted into the vagina and fitted over the cervix where it is held in place by suction. It is used with a **SPERMICIDAL** gel, cream or ointment and is a similar device to the **DIAPHRAGM**. It must not be removed for at least eight hours after intercourse and must then be washed and dried and regularly inspected for signs of wear and tear.

The cap is not suitable for a woman who has an unusually long or short cervix or one who is prone to pelvic infections. When used correctly, it has a success rate of 85 to 90 per cent but it is an unpopular method which individual women may find difficult to use. It does, however, offer some protection against **SEXUALLY TRANSMITTED DISEASES**.

DIAPHRAGM

The diaphragm is another barrier method of contraception available to women, designed to prevent the meeting of sperm and egg. It comprises a shallow, rubber dome or disc arising from a circular rim which encloses a flexible, metal ring. There are three slightly different designs and each is available in various sizes. The diaphragm must be professionally fitted and the woman given instruction as to how to insert and use it correctly.

When inserted, the diaphragm covers the whole of the cervix and fits snugly behind the pubic bone and it is used with a spermicidal preparation on either side. It can be inserted well in advance of sexual intercourse and must then be left in place for at least eight hours. It cannot be felt or dislodged by normal activity or sexual intercourse.

Like the cap, the diaphragm then needs to be removed, washed and dried, store carefully and inspected regularly for signs of damage. A regular professional check-up is required for any woman using a diaphragm and a new diaphragm is needed about every two years.

This method is used by a fairly small number of usually older women in settled relationships. If used correctly, it has a success rate of 85 to 90 per cent and it provides some measure of protection against SEXUALLY TRANSMITTED DISEASES.

FEMALE CONDOM

The female condom is a relatively new barrier method of contraception comprising a soft bag made of polyurethane which has a larger open end with a rim and a narrow blind end which is reinforced by a ring. It is much larger and stronger than the male condom. The ring at the narrow end is squeezed shut and it is then carefully inserted into the vagina using a finger. This draws most of the condom into the vagina which is correctly in place when the narrow end is beyond the pubic bone. The outer, open end remains outside the vagina and the rim of this is flattened over the vulva. After use, the outer rim is peeled off and the condom is twisted behind the rim so that it is sealed. It can then be carefully removed.

Female condoms can be bought 'over the counter' and there is no need for any medical involvement or professional fitting. However, it is advisable to practise inserting the condom as if it is not correctly placed, it may be dislodged.

The method appears to have about equal number of supporters and detractors. One of the main advantages is that failure is usually obvious, giving time for emergency contraception to be sought, and just as important, the female condom gives excellent protection against **SEXUALLY TRANSMITTED DISEASES** and infections because it covers the vulva as well as the whole of the vagina.

MALE CONDOM OR SHEATH

The male condom or sheath is a form of contraception which has a long history of use and which remains one of the two most popular methods that are currently available. A great variety of different types exist but all consist of a thin sheath, usually made or latex rubber, which is slipped onto the erect penis before penetration. The sheath adheres firmly to the skin and ejaculated sperm are passed into a 'teat' of rubber at the end of the condom. Hence the condom is a barrier method of contraception which physically prevents the meeting of sperm and egg and has a success rate of about 98 per cent, when used correctly.

Since it is, in effect, an enclosed, impermeable bag, it also affords a high degree of protection against SEXUALLY TRANSMITTED DISEASES. Problems arise if the condom slips off or is inadvertently punctured, when its effectiveness, both as a contraceptive and in protecting against infection, is obviously compromised.

Mishaps with condoms are more likely to occur in young, inexperienced males aged under 25 years and this is also the group that are least likely to use them. However, it is men in this age group who most benefit from using condoms, as they are more likely to be involved in casual sexual relationships and hence risk causing inadvertent pregnancy or picking up and/or passing on sexually transmitted diseases.

If a condom is used, the penis must be withdrawn immediately after orgasm before loss of the erection and it should be held in place to guard against the risk of it slipping off. It is important to use types which carry the BSI kite mark to ensure that they have been tested to a high standard of strength and effectiveness. A condom should not be allowed to come into contact with any chemical product that might weaken the rubber. If a lubricant is used, it should be a water-based type such as KY™ jelly which will not interfere with the composition of the condom.

SPERMICIDES

Spermicides are chemical preparations that act against sperm, either by killing or inactivating them or a combination of both. They are available in various forms – creams, foams, jellies, pessaries, etc. – for insertion into the vagina but are not a reliable contraceptive method on their own. They are mainly used in conjunction with barrier methods, such as the DIAPHRAGM, CERVICAL CAP and CONDOM, and the instructions should be carefully read to ensure that the product is suitable for this type of use.

HORMONAL CONTRACEPTIVE METHODS

Hormonal contraceptive methods use the administration of hormones, most commonly in pill form, to make the user temporarily infertile. Most are designed to be used by women but a male contraceptive pill has recently become available.

COMBINED ORAL CONTRACEPTIVE PILLS

Combined oral contraceptive pills are available in a number of different formulas which are all based on combinations of the female hormones, oestrogen and progesterone. The combined pill was first developed during the 1960s and it remains the most popular form of contraception, overall, among women. When taken correctly, it is almost entirely effective in preventing **PREGNANCY** because of the physiological effects that are produced. These include halting **OVULATION**, preventing the thickening of the **ENDOMETRIUM** so that it is not prepared to receive a fertilized egg and altering the action of the Fallopian tubes so that the passage of sperm (or egg) is not aided.

It is believed that pregnancy among pill users is usually related to some other factor, most commonly, one or more missed pills which has enabled the woman's natural cycle to be reinstated. Some prescription drugs, including antibiotics, may lower the efficacy of the combined contraceptive pill and it is thought that some women become pregnant because they do not realize that this is the case. Similarly, a bout of vomiting and/or diarrhoea may enable the hormones in the pill to be eliminated from the body before they can be absorbed. This also may result in a weakening of the effectiveness of the pill, allowing pregnancy to occur. It is important for a woman to be aware of the circumstances in which the pill might fail and to seek medical advice, if in any doubt about the effect of prescribed medicines.

The combined contraceptive pill confers a number of health benefits, including a lessening of the risk of **OVARIAN** and **ENDOMETRIAL CANCER**. It is often effective in relieving problems associated with **MENSTRUATION**, especially painful and/or heavy periods. However, the combined pill is not suitable for every woman and there are a number of medical conditions which rule out its use. Also, the pill can produce a range of side effects which include weight gain, breast tenderness, nausea, fluid retention, breakthrough bleeding and headaches. Usually, these symptoms are relatively mild and can be overcome by switching to a different product since the pill is available in varying combinations of dosage. The occurrence of side effects usually means that a particular formulation is not suitable for the individual concerned and sometimes it may be necessary to try several types before the right one is found.

Taking the pill confers a slightly higher risk of the development of heart and circulatory disorders – stroke, high blood pressure, deep vein thrombosis and pulmonary embolism – and also **BREAST CANCER**. For these reasons, it must be prescribed by a doctor (although it is available free of charge) and the woman's health monitored from time to time. Usually, there is no adverse effect upon **FERTILITY** although it may take a little time for regular cycles to be reinstated once the pill is discontinued.

PROGESTERONE-ONLY OR MINI-PILL

As its name suggests, the progesterone-only or mini-pill for women is a hormonal contraceptive pill which contains only synthetic progesterone and no oestrogen at all. Although it may prevent **OVULATION**, its main effect is upon the consistency of cervical mucus which is rendered thick and inhospitable to sperm. It also affects the activity of the Fallopian tubes, which no longer aid the passage of sperm or egg and it prevents the **ENDOMETRIUM** from thickening, so making it less able to receive a fertilized egg. The mini-pill contains a lower dose of progesterone than in any of the combined preparations and it produces fewer side effects. Although some medical conditions, such as certain cancers, circulatory disorders and previous **ECTOPIC PREGNANCY** exclude its use, it can often be taken by women for whom the combined pill is contraindicated. The mini-pill can be used by women who are **BREASTFEEDING**.

Side effects which do occur are mostly short-lived but the most common one is irregular bleeding. Others include weight gain, **LOSS OF LIBIDO**, breast tenderness, headaches, **OVARIAN CYSTS**, hair growth and acne – all generally short-lived. In the event of pill failure, there is a slightly higher risk of **ECTOPIC PREGNANCY**.

The mini-pill is highly effective if used correctly, but it must be taken at the same time each day and not more than three hours late. Hence it is only suitable for those who are entirely committed to its use. It is less popular than the combined pill and some women use it in conjunction with a barrier method of contraception.

HORMONAL CONTRACEPTIVE INJECTION

The hormonal contraceptive injection is available to women and consists of delivering a slow-release dose of synthetic progesterone (progestogen) by injection. A higher dose of progestogen is released at first and then a lower, slow-release of the hormone continues to be effective for 2 or 3 months. The hormone works in the same way as when it is taken in pill form and provides an effective method of contraception.

It is not suitable for all women and a number of medical conditions and disorders, such as heart and circulatory disease, rule out its use. It may produce certain side effects but also has a number of advantages, including the fact that the woman can forget about contraception until the next injection is due. However, if the woman decides that she wishes to become pregnant, it may take some time for regular cycles to be reinstated and for the effects of the hormone to wear off.

HORMONAL IMPLANTS

Hormonal implants is a method of contraception available to women which consists of implanting minute, plastic rods containing synthetic progesterone (progestogen) beneath the skin. Usually, 6 rods are implanted in a fan-shaped pattern, just beneath the skin of the inner, upper arm. These then slowly release a measured dose of progestogen over a period of 5 years. The implant provides effective contraception but with the same possible side effects and contraindications as other progesterone-only methods. Its advantages are that contraception does not need to be thought about for five years. However, if the woman wishes to become pregnant, fertility is restored more or less immediately once the implants are removed. Disadvantages include the necessity of having the implants inserted and removed surgically. A woman can usually feel the implants herself but they are not normally visible externally. However, some women do produce scar tissue around the site of the implant or scarring may occur upon removal.

MALE HORMONAL PILL

For many years, research has been carried out with the aim of developing an effective contraceptive pill for men which would need to work by stopping the production and/or release of sperm. This goal has proved to be an elusive one, made more difficult by the fact that millions of sperm are produced continually throughout life and so a man is normally fertile all the time. This is in marked contrast to the situation in women in whom a single egg is normally released and **FERTILITY** is restricted to a period of about 8 days in each monthly cycle. Hence, not only is it relatively simple to override a woman's fertility by means of hormonal control but also fine adjustments in dosage make it possible to achieve this with very few side effects.

Achieving a similar goal in men has appeared to be out of reach until very recently. Even when the administration of hormones (or other drugs) was able to cause a reduction in sperm production in experimental animals, undesirable side effects were very often noted. However, in the year 2000, researchers at the Centre for Reproductive Biology at Edinburgh University announced that they had achieved a breakthrough. They have formulated a hormonal contraceptive system for men which, in clinical trials carried out in Scotland and China, halted sperm production in the participants but produced no adverse effects. The pill contained a synthetic steroid hormone called desogestrel which acted on the pituitary gland of the brain, stopping it from releasing the hormones which normally stimulate testosterone and sperm production in the testicles. At the same time, the men were given a hormonal implant beneath the skin (similar to those available to women) containing testosterone in order to maintain a normal level of male hormones. After several weeks, the pill caused the participant's sperm counts to fall to zero while the implant ensured that normal masculine characteristics were maintained.

When the system was discontinued, sperm production rapidly returned to normal and several of the trial participants have since fathered children so fertility was not adversely affected. It is expected that this contraceptive system will be available commercially in about five years' time and surveys suggest that it will prove popular with men. About 60 per cent of those sampled indicated their willingness to use the system and welcomed its development.

INTRAUTERINE DEVICE (IUD)

The intrauterine device (IUD) is usually composed of inert synthetic polypropylene or polyethylene and copper wire, which is inserted into the womb. IUDs come in a variety of shapes, including that of a 7 or a T in profile, and are attached to two strong, fine threads. The device is inserted in a flattened form via a hollow tube which is passed through the cervix and it opens out once it is in place. The threads project from the IUD through the cervix and into the upper part of the

169

vagina and are used for the eventual removal of the device. Insertion of an IUD must be carried out by an experienced doctor and can be uncomfortable or even slightly painful, although the event is short-lived. Immediately following insertion, the woman may experience slight bleeding or cramps and occasionally, the IUD may be expelled altogether. Hence it is vital that the woman checks that the device is in place by feeling for the threads and this should be carried out on a weekly basis.

The contraceptive IUD may cause heavier and more painful periods (**MENORRHAGIA** but *see also* the **PROGESTOGEN-RELEASING IUD** below). Its presence makes it easier for infectious agents to gain access to the womb and higher reproductive organs and it is not suitable for women who have many sexual partners. The IUD is particularly associated with an increased risk of **PELVIC INFLAMMATORY DISEASE** and should not be used by a woman who has a previous history of **SEXUALLY TRANSMITTED INFECTION**.

Its use is also associated with a slightly increased risk of **ECTOPIC PRECNANCY** and hence is not suitable for any woman who has previously had this condition. Other medical conditions which rule out its use include existing menorrhagia or **FIBROIDS, ENDOMETRIOSIS,** anaemia, heart disease, diabetes or any circumstance in which the immune system is suppressed. Rarely, the lining of the womb may be provoked into growing and attempting to envelop the IUD so that the device starts to become embedded. In the event of this occurring, surgical removal is necessary. More rarely still and usually as a result of inept positioning, the IUD may puncture the womb and stray into the abdominal cavity. In these highly unusual circumstances, surgery is once again needed in order to remove the device.

The IUD is the third most popular form of contraception in the UK, used by around 7 to 8 per cent of women, and it can be left in place for five years. It has a success rate of 98 per cent and is believed to work by preventing the implantation of a fertilized egg. If pregnancy does occur, there is a slightly increased risk of **MISCARRIAGE** or **PREMATURE BIRTH** although the IUD itself causes no harm to the developing foetus. Removal of an IUD also increases the risk of miscarriage and so the decision whether or not to proceed has to be carefully assessed and depends upon the position of the device and the stage of the pregnancy.

PROGESTOGEN-RELEASING IUD

The progestogen-releasing IUD is a relatively new development which not only provides a highly effective means of contraception but also lacks most of the drawbacks of the older type of IUD. It combines the anti-implantation aspect of the IUD with the hormonal effects of synthetic progesterone – in this case, Levonorgestrel™, a progestogen. The IUD contains a low dose of slow release progestogen which sometimes prevents ovulation but also acts on the cervical mucus and creates an environment that is hostile to sperm. This IUD is not associated with increased risks from **SEXUALLY TRANSMITTED DISEASES** or **PELVIC INFLAMMATORY DISEASE** or **ECTOPIC PREGNANCY**. It can be used by many women for whom the conventional IUD is unsuitable, produces few or no side effects in the majority of users and is additionally now being prescribed as a treatment method for **MENOR-RHAGIA**. Critically, the progestogen-releasing IUD greatly lessens bleeding or even halts it altogether and so it is highly suitable for women who normally have heavy periods. The device can produce the side effects associated with progestogen and discomfort or pain may be experienced during insertion but, once in place, it can be left for five years, with periodic checks to ensure that all is well.

'EMERGENCY' OR POST-COITAL CONTRACEPTION (THE 'MORNING AFTER' PILL)

Two forms of post-coital contraception are available, after the event, to a woman who has had unprotected sexual intercourse or who has reason to believe that the usual method has failed. These are the so-called 'morning-after' pill and the IUD. The morning-after pill is misleadingly named in that it is effective if started within 72 hours of sexual intercourse. However, it is more effective in preventing pregnancy if started sooner, rather than later, so a woman who requires the pill should obtain it as promptly as possible. It consists of a specially formulated dose of combined oral contraceptive pills, but containing a higher level of oestrogen than is normally given. The pack contains two pills and the first must be taken within the 72 hour period following intercourse but preferably much sooner. The second is taken exactly 12 hours later.

Since the pills contain relatively high doses of hormones, they may produce side effects, especially nausea and even vomiting. If vomiting occurs within three hours of swallowing the pill, a doctor should be consulted because a further dose may be required. The pills should not be taken on an empty stomach as this increases the risk of vomiting. The morning after pill can be taken by women who would not normally be prescribed oral contraceptives because of the presence of some risk factor. This is due to the fact that although it is a high dosage formulation, its effect is short-lived and it is safe as long as it is only used rarely.

For this reason and somewhat controversially, it is now available as an over-the-counter preparation from selected pharmacies. A woman obtaining the pills in this way will, however, receive advice from a qualified pharmacist. As before, the preparation can also be obtained free of charge from family doctors, family planning clinics and hospital genital-urinary outpatient clinics. The pill works by preventing the implantation of any fertilized egg and effectiveness varies between 95 to 98 per cent but some apparent failures may be due to women being already, unknowingly, pregnant. In this event, there is no evidence that the preparation is harmful to a developing foetus.

A second form of emergency contraception available to women is the IUD which must be inserted within five days of intercourse. The IUD must be fitted by a doctor in the usual way but there should not be any difficulty in arranging this on an emergency basis. Once in place, the IUD works in the manner previously described and it is probably the best option for women who wish to continue with this form of contraception. The IUD has a higher rate of success in preventing pregnancy following unprotected intercourse than the morning after pill, being almost 100 per cent effective.

STERILISATION – MALE AND FEMALE

Sterilisation is a surgical means of obtaining permanent contraception because those who undergo it effectively become sterile. It should be treated as a permanent and non-reversible method of contraception. This is the case even though it is becoming increasingly popular for some people who have undergone the procedure to later seek to have their FERTILITY restored.

The sterilisation operation is much simpler for men than for women but anyone considering this procedure needs to give it careful thought. Sterilisation offers no protection against **SEXUALLY TRANSMITTED DISEASES** and so methods of **SAFE SEX** may still be required.

Male sterilisation – vasectomy

The sterilisation operation in men is called vasectomy because it involves severing the vas deferens on either side. It is best suited to men in settled, permanent relationships who have already had children and are certain that their family is complete. However, it may be performed on younger, childless men who have received counselling and who fully understand the implications of the operation.

Vasectomy is usually performed at an outpatient clinic and the man can return home after the procedure, which is carried out using local anaesthetic. The patient is usually asked to shave off scrotal hair and the skin is then thoroughly cleansed with an antiseptic solution. Local anaesthetic is injected under the scrotal skin and when the area is numb, two very small incisions are made on either side to expose the vasa deferentia. A short section of each vas deferens is cut out and removed and the ends are folded back on themselves and secured with stitches. Finally, the incisions in the skin are drawn together with temporary stitches that do not need to be removed and the wound is dressed. A scrotal support and well-fitting underpants can be worn to lessen any swelling.

The patient can return home immediately but should avoid any activity which might jeopardize healing or cause injury. Ordinary painkillers such as paracetamol should be sufficient to control minor discomfort or pain. Showers or baths can be resumed the day after surgery as can work, provided that this does not involve strenuous physical activity. It is rare for there to be any complications following vasectomy other than the possibility of wound infection which can follow any surgery. In the first few days, there may be minor wound pain, slight swelling and bruising but this should soon subside. Continued pain, heat and swelling probably indicates the presence of infection and medical attention should be sought. A course of antibiotics normally clears this up very quickly. Usually, vasectomy wounds are completely healed after about ten days with, at most, minute residual scarring.

Vasectomy has no effect on LIBIDO, SEXUAL PERFOR-MANCE or ORGASM and sexual relations can be resumed once healing is complete. Some men experience slight pain on orgasm for the first few times after surgery but this is usually minor and temporary. The testes continue to produce sperm but these are eventually reabsorbed since they cannot now pass along the severed vasa deferentia. Semen continues to be ejacu-lated but this contains no sperm. However, in the first few weeks following vasectomy, it is vital to use additional **CONTRACEPTION** because some sperm remain in the reproductive tract beyond the point where the vasa deferentia were cut. Detailed advice about this is always given to any man undergoing vasectomy. After a period of weeks, the man may be asked to provide a sample of semen so that it can be examined in the laboratory to ensure that it is free from sperm. Vasectomy is a popular and effective procedure which is essentially risk-free and should not cause any future physical problems.

Female sterilisation

Female sterilisation comprises surgery to seal the Fallopian tubes, either by cutting, clipping, cauterization or severing by laser. This prevents an egg released from an ovary from passing down the Fallopian tubes to the womb. It equally prevents the upward passage of sperm and so there is no possibility of sperm and egg meeting or of **FERTILIZATION** and implantation. The procedure is carried out under a general anaesthetic and usually requires an overnight stay in hospital. It is generally carried out with the aid of laparoscopy which involves the use of a special instrument called a laparoscope. This consists of a narrow, illuminated tube with a magnifying capability which is inserted via a small incision made in the region of the navel. Carbon dioxide gas is first introduced into the abdomen to dilate it and make the pelvic organs highly visible. Once the laparoscope is inserted fine instruments are introduced via a second small incision and the Fallopian tubes are sealed by one of the methods described above. Occasionally, a larger incision may be needed or less commonly, sterilisation may be carried out via a small cut through the higher vaginal wall. Following the procedure, the incisions are repaired with clips or sutures which may need to be removed later.

The woman may be able to return home on the same day once the effects of the anaesthetic have worn off. She should rest and not resume vigorous activities until recovery is complete but advice is given about this at the time of surgery. Some women experience cramping, period-type pains and/or abdominal tenderness following surgery. Referred pain is frequently felt in the shoulders caused by trapped, residual pockets of gas, but this gradually subsides. The wounds normally heal well but pain, redness and heat may indicate the presence of infection for which antibiotic treatment may be required and so medical advice should be sought.

Sterilisation is best suited to women who have had children and who are sure that their family is complete. It is not likely to be offered to childless women under the age of 25 years, who may regret the decision at a later date, unless they can put forward a very convincing argument for the operation. There may be medical reasons for sterilisation, for instance, if the woman is the carrier of a genetically transmitted disorder and has taken the decision to remain child-less. Any woman considering sterilisation will receive full counselling and should take time to think carefully about all the implications before she decides to proceed.

SAFE SEX

'Safe sex' is a concept that has mainly been developed since the advent of the Human Immunodefiency Virus (HIV) and Acquired Immune Deficiency Syndrome (AIDS) and one that has been promoted by successive governments and those working in the field of health education. In spite of widespread public discussion and media attention, there is still some confusion about what safe sex actually means. Even more worry-ingly, there is growing evidence that young people in particular, are failing to practise safe sex and so are putting their health at risk.

The aim of safe sex is to provide protection from **SEXUALLY TRANSMITTED DISEASES/INFECTIONS** while ideally, at the same time, preventing unwanted and unplanned **PREGNANCY**. The obvious way to try and achieve this is through **CONTRACEPTION** but, in fact, there is no single contraceptive method currently available that completely fulfils both roles. As has been seen, methods which are virtually foolproof in preventing pregnancy provide no protection at all against infection.

Those which offer some protection against both infection and pregnancy are the barrier methods and, of these, it is only the male and female CONDOMS that are effective. Since the female condom is not in widespread use, the male condom is the main contraceptive line of defence in the practice of safe sex. When it works properly and is used correctly, the male condom is highly effective. However, whether through human error or not, condoms sometimes burst or slip off and if this occurs, the protective effect is, of course, removed. While emergency contraception can be used in these circumstances to prevent pregnancy, an infection, the presence of which is often unsuspected, can readily be passed on. Hence safe sex should perhaps more accurately be called 'safer sex' but it remains the best means of safeguarding health.

As mentioned above, the advent of HIV/AIDS forced people to think anew about their use of condoms, such was the level of fear which was generated by this apparently new and deadly viral infection. Even though the classic (venereal) diseases (i.e. SYPHILIS and GONOR-RHOEA) which have seemingly always plagued mankind can be individually devastating, they aroused less anxiety, partly because effective antibiotics were available to treat them.

The discussions that arose as a result of HIV/AIDS also focused upon sexual behaviour and personal responsibility for safeguarding health. The seemingly carefree, sexually liberated, 'sleep around' attitudes of the 60s and 70s, which had arisen with the availability of the contraceptive pill, looked set to disappear. Instead, people were encouraged to avoid frequent, casual sexual relationships (in addition to always using condoms). This behavioural aspect of safe sex remains just as relevant today and lies within the choice of each individual.

General anxiety about HIV infection (or any other **SEXUALLY TRANSMITTED DISEASE**) has, rightly or wrongly, declined in Western countries where treatment is available. Recent surveys in Britain confirm that those who are most at risk of acquiring a sexually transmitted infection (and/or having an unplanned pregnancy) are teenagers and young adults. But in spite of the widespread availability of information and sex education, this is the very age group which is least likely to be concerned or to practise any form of safe sex. Accompanying this lack of concern, there has been an alarming explosion in the incidence of teenage pregnancies and sexually transmitted diseases – particularly **CHLAMYDIA** which, it appears, many people are unaware of (*see* next chapter). Alerting young people to the health risks which they face and persuading them to change their behaviour and practise safe sex, remains one of the most important challenges facing Britain today. (*See also* Chapter 12.)

CHAPTER 11

Sexually transmitted diseases (STDs) and infections

Sexually transmitted diseases are diseases that are usually acquired through sexual intercourse and they are very common and sometimes extremely severe in their effects. Several STDs can be passed on through anal and oral sex as well as by vaginal intercourse. Others included in this section, in addition to being passed on sexually, can be acquired through inoculation with infected blood or body fluid.

Some STDs cause early symptoms in the genital region which alert the sufferer to the possibility of infection but others, unfortunately, do not. Symptoms may be produced in people of one gender and not the other which can make it difficult both to treat and halt the spread of the infection. Even where early symptoms are produced, some individuals may not experience them or they may be so slight that they remain unnoticed. This situation can be very dangerous as very often the infection is then able to spread to the internal reproductive organs where it may cause irreversible damage, possibly leading to **INFERTILITY**. In the meantime, the person harbouring the STD may also unknowingly be infecting others.

Anyone who suspects the presence of an infection should seek medical advice, either through a GP or at a genito-urinary clinic run by most of the larger general hospitals. All doctors' surgeries have leaflets and posters, usually prominently displayed, giving details about where and when genito-urinary clinics are held in their local area. A phone number is always available, making it simple to obtain the necessary information about when to attend. Hence anyone who is sensitive about consulting his or her own GP can readily obtain confidential diagnosis and treatment. Doctors at a GU clinic are experts in this area of medicine and patients can expect to obtain an accurate diagnosis and suitable treatment and advice.

Usually, a physical examination is carried out and a swab obtained of any discharge so that organisms can be cultured. The person will be asked about other symptoms, may be asked to give details about his or her sexual activities, but only if this is relevant to the diagnosis. Results and treatment, normally in the form of the most appropriate antibiotics, are available very swiftly. Follow-up appointments will usually be arranged until the infection has been completely eradicated. The clinic will also wish to get in touch with the person's sexual partner(s) so that they too can receive advice and treatment. This is carried out without revealing the identity of the original patient. A person may be reluctant to disclose information out of a misguided sense of shame or embarrassment. However, it is important to remember that STDs can have severe consequences and it is selfish to leave someone else at risk. Also, anyone who has an STD acquired it, in the first place, from someone else and embarrassment is one of the reasons why these diseases are able to spread so readily. It is much better to break a chain of infection and ensure that people are treated when necessary even at the risk of some initial upset.

CHLAMYDIA TRACHOMATIS

Chlamydia, as it is usually known, is a sexually transmitted disease caused by a strange bacterium that resembles a virus in its habits, in that it lives inside human cells and is dependent upon them for its growth and replication. Hence it has some characteristics of a parasite and it is commonly found in the vagina and cervix of women and in the urethra and urinary tract of people of both sexes. It can also inhabit the rectum, eyes, liver, mouth, throat and lungs, usually living within epithelial (lining) cells.

Former diagnostic techniques often failed to detect chlamydia but advances in testing have revealed that the infection is widespread and rising. There are upwards of 170,000 new cases each year in the UK alone and this highly infectious organism is easily transmitted from one person to another. Unfortunately for women, in whom the infection is most damaging, chlamydia produces no symptoms in about 70 per cent of those who are infected. Hence it is frequently unsuspected and untreated and may then move up the reproductive tract, possibly causing **CERVICITIS**, salpingitis (inflammation and infection of the **FALLOPIAN TUBES**) and **PELVIC INFLAMMATORY DISEASE**.

These infections may not be detected until irrevocable damage has been caused to the Fallopian tubes. Sometimes, a woman may only discover what has happened when she seeks treatment for **INFERTILITY**. Even when a woman does develop early symptoms of chlamydia infection, which may include a more profuse vaginal discharge and frequent and painful urination, they are easily confused with other infections such as cystitis. The spread of the infection to the higher reproductive organs can be aided by having gynaecological procedures (such as a D and C) or being fitted with, or having an existing, IUD. The presence of chlamydia confers a greater risk of **ECTOPIC PREGNANCY** and during a normal pregnancy, there is a greater likelihood of **MISCARRIAGE, PREMATURE DELIVERY** and **STILLBIRTH**.

About half of the babies born to chlamydia-infected mothers acquire the infection themselves during delivery. Most commonly, the newborn develops a type of conjunctivitis when about one week old. However, up to 20 per cent of infants may develop pneumonia as a result of the infection, usually some weeks after birth, posing a serious health risk. Both these conditions can be treated but worryingly, chlamydia is associated with a greater risk of sudden death in the weeks after birth. Labour and delivery provide a further opportunity for chlamydia to spread and a new mother with an unsuspected infection is at greater risk of developing **PELVIC INFLAMMATORY DISEASE.**

Recent studies have revealed that chlamydia is responsible for at least half of all cases of what was formerly called non-specific urethritis in men. Chlamydia infection in men usually causes symptoms (although 10 per cent of infected men remain symptom-free). The usual symptoms are a clear or yellowish discharge from the penis and a slight, prickling discomfort or mild burning sensation during urination. The symptoms usually occur within one to four weeks of infection and any man who notices them should seek medical advice and treatment. If left, the infection may spread to the testicles causing much more severe symptoms of pain, heat, swelling and fever. In both men and women, the organism may gain access to the rectum or, less commonly, be transferred to the eyes and cause conjunctivitis.

Treatment is both simple and effective once a

diagnosis has been made and consists of oral doses of appropriate antibiotics. It is essential for all sexual partners to be treated and this is especially important in the case of chlamydia which can quietly be causing damage without making its presence felt.

TRICHOMONIASIS

Trichomoniasis is an infection caused by a single-celled, protozoal, micro-organism that is larger than bacteria or viruses and is called Trichomonas vaginalis. It is a common inhabitant of the rectum in both men and women where it causes no harm. However, if it gets into the vagina it causes irritation, inflammation and itching, along with a greenish discharge which has a fish-like odour. It may also spread to the urethra and cause symptoms of cystitis (i.e. frequent, painful urination with a burning sensation).

In men, trichomonas can inhabit the warm, damp area beneath the foreskin and can also survive for a time within the urethra, although this is usually short-lived. It may produce no symptoms but if these do arise, they include a discoloured, greenish discharge and slight pelvic pain. Rarely, the organism may spread to the prostate gland and exceptionally, it may then generate cystitis-like symptoms. Trichomonas is most commonly spread by sexual contact but it may gain access from the rectum if it is present there. Although the organism is generally short-lived in men and often symptom-free, a man can easily pass the infection on to other sexual partners. Rarely, the organism is acquired from the environment, for example from a contaminated towel.

In **PREGNANCY**, trichomonas confers a greater risk of a **PREMATURE BIRTH** and it is possible that it may be acquired by a baby during birth itself, possibly causing respiratory infections. Treatment is by means of a course of an antimicrobial drug such as metronidazole and sexual partners should also be treated to avoid reinfection.

GENITAL HERPES

Herpes is an extremely common virus and occurs most frequently in two forms, herpes simplex virus 1 (HSV 1) and herpes simplex virus 2 (HSV 2). HSV 1 is the virus which causes cold sores in some people, but it is believed that many others acquire the organism but it then remains dormant in a nerve root and does not manifest itself. HSV2 is a closely related strain of the virus which causes genital herpes alone. However, it is now known that HSV 1 can also cause genital herpes and is responsible for a varying proportion of all cases. In this case, it is contracted by having oral sex with a person who has an active cold sore.

Genital herpes is common, contagious and often very painful, although severity of attacks vary between individuals and tends to lessen with the passage of time. Once acquired, the virus cannot be eliminated from the body and although symptoms and frequency of attacks can be alleviated by drug treatments, the condition can have a considerable impact upon normal life. The description that follows applies to a severe attack of genital herpes.

Usually, there is an early indication that the condition is about to erupt, known as the prodromal sign. This varies but may take the form of mild irritation in the genital region or slight pain or discomfort, which may also occur in the pelvic area and/or upper thighs. This is followed by the eruption of clear, fluid-filled blisters which usually occur about one week after initial infection. These blisters occur on the vulva and perineum in women and anywhere on the external genitals in men. They may also arise internally on mucous membranes including those lining the anus. The blisters eventually burst, turn yellow and crust over, signalling that the attack is coming to an end but the sufferer can experience extreme pain before this stage is reached. There may be accompanying symptoms of fever, malaise, headaches, swollen lymph glands in the groin and a burning sensation on passing urine. The latter symptom is caused by urine coming into contact with the blisters.

A first attack of genital herpes is usually more prolonged and produces the most severe symptoms which may last for two to three weeks. Subsequent outbreaks, if they occur at all, range in frequency and severity between individuals. About half of those affected never experience another attack, others only a few, while a minority experience an outbreak every two or three months. Drugs are available to help those who are more severely affected but in all cases, the condition generally improves with time.

Treatment is by means of antiviral drugs, particularly Acyclovir™ or Zovirax™ but newer ones are also being developed. Medication may be given both orally (i.e. by mouth) and/or topically (i.e. as cream or ointment applied directly to sores). Bed rest and analgesia may help to relieve the other symptoms which may accompany an attack. Usually, drug treatment is only necessary for the first occurrence of genital herpes and any subsequent attack can be managed by self-help measures.

These include bathing the sores in tepid water containing a little dissolved salt to encourage healing, taking cool baths or showers to relieve pain and wearing breathable cotton underwear and avoiding tight-fitting trousers. It is essential to seek early medical advice and treatment for a first attack of genital herpes. Sexual intercourse must be avoided while any signs or blisters are present, until healing is complete and would, in any case, be very painful. Anyone with a cold sore should be careful until the lesion has healed, as this is the time when HSV can be passed on. The virus can survive in the environment for a time and so it is important not to share towels and flannels and to be scrupulous about personal hygiene.

The use of condoms offers the best protection against infection and the virus is only likely to be passed on during an active attack. A first attack of genital herpes during childbirth is dangerous for the baby who will usually become infected. There is a serious risk of death or severe impairment in these circumstances. A mother who harbours the virus will have produced antibodies which will usually be passed to the baby during development. An expectant mother with a history of recurrent attacks of genital herpes will usually be delivered by **CAESAREAN SECTION** to avoid any risks to her baby.

The herpes virus can also cause eye infection – a form of conjunctivitis that may lead to ulceration and scarring of the cornea and even to loss of vision. This is much more likely to arise as a result of the virus being transferred from a cold sore to the eye on a finger, but it can occur in the same way with genital herpes. Hence it is necessary to be scrupulous about hand-washing during an attack of genital herpes and to immediately seek medical attention for any symptoms of eye infection. Genital herpes which affects the **CERVIX** in women is one of the risk factors associated with **CERVICAL CANCER**. Hence a woman who has had an attack of herpes in this region may require more frequent **CERVICAL SMEAR TESTS** than is usual as a protective measure.

GENITAL WARTS

Many warts are caused by strains of human papilloma virus (HPV) and genital warts are no exception. In both men and women, genital warts can occur externally on the surface of the genitalia or around the anus. They may also occur internally, within the rectum or urethra and in the vagina and on the cervix in women. If the warts are internal, their presence may not be suspected for some time. The warts may occur either singly or clustered in groups, appearing as small, pinkish-red irregular bumps or they may be flat. Internal, flat wars are often only detected by specialized diagnostic techniques. Genital warts usually appear between one and six months after infection but produce few or no symptoms. Slight itching or irritation may be noticed and women may have a more profuse discharge than is usual. The latter is not caused by the warts themselves but provides an ideal environment in which they can thrive and grow. Genital warts are found in warm, moist situations and so conditions which create this favour their proliferation. They can rarely occur in the mouth when the route of infection is oral sex.

Anyone who suspects the presence of genital warts should seek immediate medical advice and treatment.

Treatment usually takes the form of applications of a solution of podophyllin or other preparation to kill the warts. Alternatively, they may be removed by cryosurgery, laser, cauterisation or conventional surgery under local anaesthetic. Genital warts can be quite persistent and often recur so treatment may need to be continued for some time.

There is an established link between infection with certain strains of HPV and the occurrence of precancerous changes in the **CERVIX** and **CSRVICAL CANCER** in women. In particular, HPV is associated with a more aggressive form of the disease that has emerged in younger women and which is on the increase. The emergence and rise in the number of such cases has to a certain extent been linked with an increased incidence of genital warts. However, infection with other strains of the human papilloma virus can be asymptomatic, i.e. without the presence of genital warts but still acquired through sexual contact. The HPV virus has been detected in many abnormal cervical smear tests where cells are showing signs of precancerous changes. However, it should be emphasized that HPV infection is one among a number of risk factors and does not mean that a woman is inevitably going to develop cervical cancer. A woman who has had HPV infection/genital warts may be advised to have an annual cervical smear test instead of one every three years. Sexual partners should also receive treatment and an infected man must use condoms to limit the risk of transmitting the virus.

GONORRHOEA

Gonorrhoea is a common STD which can also (but rarely) be contracted through contact with an infective discharge on towels, flannels, bedding, etc. The causative micro-organism is a bacterium called Neisseria gonorrhoeae which is highly infectious and invades mucous membranes. In women, it is found mainly in the vagina and cervix and, less commonly, in the urethra, rectum and throat. In men, it is found in the urethra and sometimes in the rectum and throat. Oral sex is responsible for infection of the throat.

In **HOMOSEXUAL** and **BISEXUAL** men, anal sex is the means of infection of rectal tissues. In women, the organism may find its way into the rectum due to the close proximity of the vaginal opening and the anus. Unprotected sex with an infected person carries a high risk (90 per cent) of infection and gonorrhoea is the most prevalent STD in the world.

Most men develop symptoms within one to two weeks of infection and these are a thick, yellowish discharge of pus from the penis and pain which may be intense when urinating. If the throat is infected, it may become sore and inflamed with a discharge of pus. Likewise, if the rectum is involved, there may be inflammation with a discharge from the anus. About

20 per cent of men have lesser or milder symptoms.

In women, the positions are reversed with about 80 per cent experiencing no symptoms or ones which are so slight as to avoid notice. This situation is particularly dangerous as it enables the organism to spread and cause damage to the reproductive organs. If symptoms do occur, they may include a slight discharge which may be discoloured and discomfort with urination. Or, there may be a sore throat or inflammation of the rectum, if these areas are infected.

If not diagnosed and treated promptly, gonorrhoea can spread and cause irreversible damage in as little as eight to ten weeks. In women, the Fallopian tubes are particularly vulnerable with possible inflammation, infection and blockage and the risk of INFERTILITY and ECTOPIC PREGNANCY. At this stage, the woman is likely to have experienced symptoms of PELVIC INFLAMMATORY DISEASE such as low back pain, fever and painful, heavy periods. A rare complication is potentially fatal peritonitis. In men, the TESTICLES and PROSTATE GLAND may be infected which may affect fertility. If the urethra is involved and there is prolonged inflammation, there is a risk of stricture due to the formation of scar tissue.

In the longer term, further complications can arise in both sexes, especially if gonorrhoea remains untreated. These include inflammation of the eyes (conjunctivitis), joints (gonococcal arthritis), heart valves (endocarditis) and blood poisoning (septicaemia).

Gonorrhoea affecting the cervix poses a risk during childbirth as the baby is likely to contract the infection during its passage down the birth canal. The baby's eyes are especially vulnerable and the infant develops swollen, discharging eyes within two days of birth. The infection must be treated promptly with antibiotics or there is a risk of permanent impairment or loss of vision. Until comparatively recently, this condition, known as ophthalmia neonatorum, was a major cause of infant blindness and it continues to pose a threat in circumstances where medical treatment is lacking.

Anyone who suspects that they may have contracted gonorrhoea should seek immediate medical advice. Diagnosis is made by taking a swab of any discharge and culturing the organism. Treatment is usually very effective when received promptly and is in the form of oral doses of antibiotics, normally penicillin, tetracycline or sulphonamides.

Follow-up tests are carried out for a time to make sure that the bacteria have been completely eradicated. If there have been any complications, these may require further treatment depending upon the extent of the problem. Condom use provides the best means of avoiding infection.

SYPHILIS

Syphilis is an infectious STD caused by the bacterium Treponema paldium which is known as the treponeme.

The full course of the disease occurs in three stages and takes months or even years to develop. Before the advent of modern antibiotic treatments, syphilis was a feared disease and a cause of early death, but its worst manifestations can now, fortunately, be prevented. However, it remains a serious health risk, especially for people who do not have access to good medical care.

The bacteria enter the body through minute tears in mucous membranes and are transmitted during unprotected sexual intercourse with an infected person. Membranes lining the rectum are thin and easily damaged so that people who engage in anal sex are at greater risk of infection. In men, the site of infection is usually the penis or anus and in women, the vaginal and urethral openings, clitoris and sometimes the cervix. The mouth may become infected if the bacteria have entered during oral sex. The first symptom is the appearance of a painless ulcer called a chancre at the site of infection, which usually appears after about two weeks but may take up to three months to develop. Within a short time the lymph nodes enlarge and harden, first locally near the site of the infection and then all over the body and this stage lasts for several weeks. The primary chancre usually heals during this period.

If the person remains untreated, secondary stage symptoms appear about two months after initial infection and may overlap with the first stage. Usually a rash of red spots appears which may be noticed at first on the chest but may occur almost anywhere. Also, there is malaise, aches and pains in muscles and joints, fever, anorexia, swollen lymph glands and tiredness as by this stage the disease involves the whole body. There may even be hair loss and enlargement of the liver but eventually, symptoms may subside and enter a resting phase. Infective bacteria are present in enormous numbers in both the primary chancre and any secondary stage skin lesions and a person with untreated syphilis is infective for a prolonged period.

Tertiary or 3rd stage syphilis is rare in modern medicine and even if syphilis is not treated, does not always appear. It occurs months or years after initial infection and only in untreated people. Numerous tumour-like masses form throughout the body in organs such as the skin, muscles, bones, liver, stomach, brain and spinal cord and cause severe damage. Blindness, paralysis, dementia, heart failure and early death may all be consequences of tertiary syphilis.

Congenital syphilis can be passed on from an infected mother to her unborn child via the placenta with very serious consequences for the baby. In Western countries, this is very rare as expectant mothers are screened routinely for the presence of syphilis by means of a blood sample which is checked for the presence of the organism. Anyone who suspects that he (or she) may have been infected with syphilis should seek immediate medical advice. A swab is taken from a lesion to confirm diagnosis and treatment is then simple and effective, comprising a course of antibiotics, usually penicillin. (Alternatives are available to treat those who are adversely affected by penicillin.) Prompt treatment avoids the development of second stage symptoms and follow-up tests ensure that the organism has been eradicated.

HEPATITIS B (HBV)

Also known as serum hepatitis B, hepatitis B (HBV) is a serious and potentially fatal form of liver disease which is usually, although not solely, sexually transmitted. The causal organism is a virus which is responsible for a range of disorders and symptoms, varying from an acute attack of liver inflammation to a chronic, aggressive disease which eventually may cause cirrhosis and premature death. HBV is also associated with liver (hepato-cellular) cancer which is common in populations with a high prevalence of the virus. At the other extreme, people may be infected with HBV and subsequently eliminate the virus from the body without showing signs of illness. Or, the symptoms may be so mild that they are disregarded. About 10 per cent of those infected become chronic carriers of the virus, which can persist in the body in a dormant state for many years. These people provide a reservoir of HBV and may unknowingly infect others. They are also at a substantially greater risk of future liver disease, especially cirrhosis and cancer. Blood tests can reveal the presence of anti-HBV antibodies that indicate past exposure and infection and screening has shown that the virus is particularly prevalent among certain groups of people, although anyone can be infected.

HBV is highly infectious and exists in blood and body fluids, especially vaginal and rectal secretions, semen and saliva. The highest concentration occurs in blood. The virus is transmitted when infected blood or body fluid comes into contact with and is able to invade the tissues of a non-infected person. The virus may gain access through cuts and abrasions or by unprotected, heterosexual intercourse and/or anal and oral sex. In Western countries, all blood and blood products are screened for the presence of HBV and so transfusion poses no risk. The main route of infection involving blood is the sharing of contaminated needles by injecting drug users. Also, tattooing, ear and body piercing, acupuncture and minor dental and surgical procedures are further areas of potential risk although stringent guidelines are in place in the UK to ensure that procedures are as safe as possible.

Health care workers and those involved in the activities just listed are themselves at greater risk of infection – for example from 'needlestick' injuries. This refers to them being accidentally pierced by needles, scalpels, etc. while engaged in their work and there is an obvious potential risk for doctors and nurses who are treating a person who is bleeding. At even higher risk are those who have unprotected sex, especially with numerous sexual partners, injecting drug users, people engaged in prostitution and those who are in prison where there is a greater likelihood of drug and sexual abuse. A baby can acquire HBV from an infected mother during birth and infants of drug abusing parents are at obvious risk.

The incubation period for HBV is usually between six weeks and six months. When symptoms occur, they are typical of acute hepatitis and include headache, fever, aches, pains, chills, malaise, nausea, sickness, loss of appetite, skin rashes, painful, swollen wrists and ankles, jaundice and the passing of dark urine and pale-coloured stools. Most people make a gradual recovery, although this may take several weeks and abnormal feelings of tiredness may last for some months. A small proportion of people go on to develop chronic hepatitis which has a similar range of symptoms that may persist for years. These may eventually end in cirrhosis, liver failure and death in some of those affected. Anyone who has any symptoms of liver disease or who has reason to suspect HBV infection should seek immediate medical advice.

Diagnosis is made by analysis of blood samples for the presence of certain antigen-antibody systems which detect the presence of hepatitis B. Treatment consists of bed rest, plenty of fluids, avoidance of alcohol and analgesic pain relief. Those who develop chronic hepatitis may require hospitalisation and treatment with antiviral drugs such as interferon. The mortality rate in those who are severely affected can be quite high.

Vaccination against HBV infection is not available to everyone in the UK but is offered to health care workers and may be given to others who are at high risk. Pregnant women are routinely screened for HBV and babies considered to be at risk are vaccinated. Protection against HBV not only involves the practice of SAFE SEX but also personal lifestyle choices to limit risk. Anyone who seeks acupuncture, ear or body piercing or tattooing should ensure that the premises attended adhere to all safety guidelines, especially in the use of sterile, disposable needles. Since the virus can survive for a short time in the environment, items connected with personal hygiene such as razors, flannels, towels, etc. should not be shared with others.

HEPATITIS C (HCV)

Hepatitis C is caused by an RNA virus and was first identified in 1987. It is spread through direct contact with the blood of an infected person. The most common means of transmission is through sharing needles with infected intravenous drug users. Prior to

1990 there was no reliable way of testing donated blood for the virus and some people have become infected through receiving a blood transfusion contaminated with HCV. However, since 1990 blood for transfusions has been tested for this virus. Anyone having unprotected sex with an infected person may also be at risk of becoming infected.

In many cases, it is 20 or 30 years before the patient is found to have the infection and to date there is no vaccine capable of providing protection against HCV infection. For how to protect yourself, see the suggestions given above for HBV.

HIV/AIDS

AIDS is Acquired Immune Deficiency Syndrome which was first recognized in the USA in 1981. The causal agent was identified soon afterwards, in 1983, and designated the Human Immunodeficiency Virus. In the early years of HIV and AIDS, a huge amount of fear was generated and the epidemic brought an end to the carefree attitude to sex that had arisen during the previous 20 years with the introduction of the CONTRA-CEPTIVE PILL. (Although the pill did not and does not, of course, offer any protection against sexually transmitted diseases.)

HIV/AIDS was seen as a lethal combination and it seemed there was little that medicine could do to combat them. In Western countries, this perception had an impact upon people's sexual behaviour and the principles of safe sex were introduced and widely accepted. However, attitudes have changed again in recent years; levels of anxiety have declined and people have become accustomed to HIV and AIDS even though they are never out of the news for long. In Britain, this is partly attributable to the many other health scares that have become a new focus of concern – particularly the BSE/VCJD crisis. Also, although the numbers of people infected have been considerable, the early, doomsday predictions of deaths upon an apocalyptic scale have not been fulfilled in Western countries. And, most importantly of all, in recent years, the drug treatments for HIV infection have markedly improved.

The perception that the virus and the illnesses that it causes can be controlled has gained credence in the public mind and has reduced the level of fear. Whether this perception is justified or not is discussed in the summary at the end of this section.

HIV is a ribonucleic (RNA) retrovirus that is able to introduce its genetic material into the DNA of cells involved in the operation of the body's immune system. It causes a gradual weakening of natural immunity which allows opportunistic infections to gain hold in the body. These illnesses and diseases vary but are collectively referred to as AIDS. The virus is found in blood and body fluids – particularly semen –

but also vaginal and other secretions. The main route of infection is through sexual intercourse, both hetero-sexual and homosexual. However, it can be passed on in any circumstances where secretions containing HIV are able to gain access to the blood of a non-infected person. Once this has occurred, the virus invades cells of the immune system known as CD4+ T-lymphocytes and a quiescent period may then follow, lasting months or even years, in which the person remains well.

Usually, the virus then becomes active again, kills its host cells and invades new ones, gradually spreading throughout the immune system. The parts of the body involved are the lymph glands and nodes, bone marrow, spleen and liver. As this process occurs, the immune system is weakened and any of a range of symptoms and infections may appear. These early AIDS symptoms include enlarged and painful glands, aches, pains, chills and fever, diarrhoea, weight loss and loss of appetite, skin rashes and dermatitis, persis-tent cough, infected throat and respiratory illnesses, night sweats and THRUSH-type fungal infections in women.

Later, secondary stage serious illnesses and cancers associated with AIDS may develop which are highly debilitating and life-threatening. These include a 'wasting' syndrome, diseases of the brain and central nervous system, a form of pneumonia known as pneumocystis carinii pneumonia, Kaposi's sarcoma (rare except in AIDS) and non-Hodgkins lymphoma. The range of illnesses that are particularly associated with AIDS are known as AIDS indicator conditions. Other symptoms and infections may be called the AIDS-Related Complex or ARC.

A simple blood test can detect the presence of HIV and newer diagnostic techniques are now available which are even more accurate. HIV infection can and often is diagnosed when a person is symptomless. Much can be done to delay the onset of AIDS in terms of a healthy lifestyle and early diagnosis allows an individual to make any necessary lifestyle changes and to take measures, such as practising safe sex, to protect any sexual partners from infection. Hence anyone who fears that he or she might be infected, or who simply wants reassurance, should have an HIV blood test. This is freely available and completely confidential and can be obtained by attending a clinic run by a local hospital, where counselling should be available. There is no need to consult a GP and information about how to obtain an HIV blood test is widely available.

It is thought that a very small number of infected people have a natural immunity to HIV and do not develop AIDS symptoms. A much greater number of people are now living with the virus and, although they may have experienced illness, effective, new drug treatments are controlling symptoms and delaying, or possibly preventing, the onset of full AIDS.

HIV-positive people and people with AIDS can now be treated with 'cocktails' of several drugs including powerful antiviral agents and protease (enzyme) inhibitors. Unfortunately, such drugs can produce toxic side effects, and a certain number of patients do not respond to this treatment. These latest drug treatments are also very expensive and until recently have been out of reach of some of the people who need them most – the millions of people with AIDS in the poorest countries of the world, notably those in sub-Saharan Africa. However, recent developments mean that these countries are now able to produce generic alternatives at a much lower cost.

HIV is no respecter of persons and anyone, male or female, can become infected. Adults are usually infected through having unprotected sexual intercourse but intravenous drug users are at particular risk if contaminated needles are shared. A great effort has been made to address this problem by issuing registered addicts with sterile, disposable needles. Unfortunately, the drug habit still causes people to take risks and so gives HIV a chance to claim more victims.

Babies born to infected mothers are at risk of acquiring HIV mainly during labour and the birth process and through breast-feeding. In Western countries, access to good medical care and delivery by Caesarean section can minimize the risks to infants but children in many other parts of the world are not so fortunate. Doctors, nurses, dental and health care workers are at risk when dealing with infected blood or body secretions or from accidental 'needlestick' injuries. Strict procedures and guidelines have to be followed in all hospitals and surgeries to protect staff. Infection in the opposite direction, from a doctor, nurse or dentist with HIV to a patient, has occurred but is exceedingly rare.

Blood donations were once a means of transmission of HIV but blood and blood products are screened for the presence of the virus in all Western countries. In Britain, donors have to answer a series of detailed and searching questions about their lifestyle (in the form of a printed questionnaire) before they can give blood. Any doubts about possible exposure to HIV are revealed by this process and the person is then discreetly asked not to be a donor. The person will be advised to have an HIV blood test if he or she is thought to be at risk. The combination of voluntary questioning of donors and screening blood is a system that works well in Britain and the risk of an infected donation 'slipping through the net' is extremely small.

On an individual level, people can take sensible precautions to limit their risk of infection by using condoms and avoiding numerous, casual sexual relationships. There are now more cases of HIV infection among heterosexuals than homosexuals in Britain and the dramatic increase in other sexually transmitted diseases is of great concern since infection with any STD that causes open sores leaves the individual concerned much more vulnerable to HIV infection. Worldwide about 80 per cent of all new cases are in sub-Saharan Africa and it is in these countries that AIDS is at its most devastating. AIDS has simply removed most of the young adults on whom the economy of a country largely depends and left children orphaned, many of whom will develop the disease in their turn. It can be seen that HIV/AIDS remains a huge global problem which affects all the world's inhabitants and the war against the disease is far from being won.

On a positive note, AIDS is a preventable disease – through the practice of safe sex and using condoms which offer almost 100 per cent protection against HIV infection. Also, research scientists and pharmaceutical companies are working hard to develop vaccines and new drugs to combat the disease. An exciting breakthrough was announced in 2001 which, it is hoped, will help to curtail the spread of HIV/AIDS. Researchers in Minnesota, USA, have developed a spermicidal contraceptive gel which incorporates a microbicide that appears to prevent the HIV virus from causing harm. In Britain, the Medical Research Council are working on a similar gel containing sticky microbicidal molecules that adhere to the virus and prevent it from entering body cells.

Although condoms offer effective protection, men are not always willing to use them or may not have access to them, especially in those countries where the AIDS epidemic is at its worst. Women are put at risk of infection but often lack the status or power to insist that their menfolk use condoms. It is hoped that the gel, which can be used directly by women and will not be detectable once in place, will enable women to protect themselves and hence their children. Ideally, it is hoped that a non-contraceptive version of the gel will also be developed which will contain the protective microbicide but will also enable women to conceive if they wish to do so. The gel is not yet available but it is hoped that it will complete successful trials in the next five years and that it will then become widely available. The World Health Organisation believes that if this product proves to be as effective as early studies suggest, it will have a considerable impact upon the AIDS epidemic.

CHAPTER 12

Sex education

Britain has the highest rate of teenage pregnancy in Western Europe and very many young people under the age of 16 years (the legal 'age of consent') admit to having sexual intercourse. In all too many instances, first sexual intercourse is unprotected and young people often only start to think about **CONTRACEPTION** and **SAFE SEX** after they have become sexually active rather than before. A further cause for concern is that the rate of **SEXUALLY TRANSMITTED DISEASES** is rising at an alarming rate in young people under the age of 20 years. The rates are particularly bad for **GONORRHOEA** and **CHLAMYDIA** infections, with worrying implications for the reproductive health of the individuals concerned.

All schools throughout the United Kingdom are required to provide sex education for pupils and it is Government policy to make access to advice and contraceptive services freely available to young people. However, in spite of a great deal of concerted effort, levels of ignorance and unconcern remain high, as is reflected by the high rates of teenage pregnancy and sexually transmitted diseases. A determined effort is being made to turn this situation around and there are a great many experts working in this field. It is beyond the scope of this book to cover all aspects of the, at times, controversial, subject of sex education. However, there seems to be fairly general agreement upon certain points and these are discussed below:

1 Ideally, parents should accept and be prepared to shoulder their responsibility for educating their children about sex and relationships. Surveys overwhelmingly reveal that children themselves feel that their early sex education should come from their parents and not from school. In the teenage years, young people want to be able to discuss sexual matters with their parents but often feel inhibited from doing so. There are no hard and fast rules about how this should be achieved but good advice is to answer young children's questions honestly when they arise in a way which they are able to understand. As a child grows older, it is important to be sure that he or she understands about the changes that will take place at **PUBERTY** and the biological facts about sex. Many parents find this difficult and embarrassing but children appreciate it when the effort is made. There are booklets available which can provide a focus for discussion and perhaps make

things easier for both parents and children. Parents should always invite their children to come to them at any time with any questions or problems that they may have.

2 Telling children about the biological facts of sex is not enough on its own and is, in some senses, the easy part. Most people remain uneasy with the idea of sex being relegated to the position of just another pastime that can be freely indulged in for self-gratification alone, even though this is the view that is often promoted in the media. Hence, from Government level downwards, it is felt that sex education should also include a broader framework that encompasses relationships and acceptable codes of conduct. Once again, parents and other adults in a young person's life have a critical role to play as they know the child best and can sensitively explore the issues involved. This is a very wide subject but perhaps, at its heart, lies the need to teach young people to value themselves (and so others) and to be sensitive to their feelings and emotions. This enables them to examine all the issues involved in having early sex, including peer pressure, which, in turn, helps them to make informed choices about their sexual behaviour. Studies show that most young people under the age of 16, who have had sex, later regret it and wish that they had waited until they were older. Many feel

disillusioned and experience a loss of self-respect. Hence it is very important for young people to realize that they can say no to sex and also, that the law exists to protect those aged under 16. Girls need to be taught that early sex and many sexual partners considerably increase their risk of **CERVICAL CANCER**. Obviously, all young people need to be made aware of the need to practise **SAFE SEX** and the very great dangers to their health posed by **SEXUALLY TRANS-MITTED DISEASES**.

3 Many young people, including children aged under 16 years, are sexually active and they will continue to be so whatever the protestations of adults. Hence, in the view of most experts and as part of Government policy, it is important to provide them with readily accessible contraceptive and health advice, which is completely confidential and non-judgemental. Also, information about how to use these services and where they are located should be displayed in places frequented by young people. It is current Government policy to put into place the type of services that are specifically geared towards the needs of young people, in order to reduce the rates of teenage pregnancy and sexually transmitted infections. This is, however, a controversial policy, attracting criticism from some parents who feel that they have a right to know about all matters concerning their

children, particularly if they are underage. Opposition has also been voiced by 'pro-life' and some religious groups, especially with regard to the provision of **ABORTION** for pregnant, teenage girls.

4 In a wider context, it is important to raise the aspirations of all young people with regard to education, career and work opportunities and various measures have been introduced to try and bring this about. Schools have a critical role to play, especially for the many children whose home circumstances are far from ideal. Studies suggest that when young people are encouraged to reach their full potential, they learn to value themselves and others more highly and this has an impact upon their sexual behaviour, resulting in, for example, fewer teenage pregnancies. But it is just as important that young teenage mothers receive support and encouragement to continue with their education and fulfil their career aspirations.

5 'Parenting classes' have been introduced into some schools as part of the personal and social education curriculum. These endeavour to demonstrate what it is like to have to cope with the demands of a baby and small child and what personal and financial responsibilities are involved. Usually, the effect of these types of programmes in schools is to make

young people more determined to avoid early parent-hood and to become more responsible in their use of contraception. Educational programmes of this nature are likely to become more common in schools as part of the drive to raise awareness and to encourage responsible sexual behaviour.

6 Alcohol and drug abuse should be included in educational programmes and discussions about sexual behaviour. Surveys suggest that young people often have sex while intoxicated or 'high' on drugs. Under these circumstances, they are vulnerable and more likely to have unprotected sex. Contraception is often not thought about and the young person is open to manipulation and abuse by older adults. In the worst case scenarios, young people cannot even remember what happened the night before. Hence the link between alcohol and drug use and sexual behaviour should always be discussed so that young people are made aware of potential risks.

CHAPTER 13

Planning conception

Many women and their partners continue to believe
that having a baby is simply a matter of ceasing to use
contraception and that **PREGNANCY** will be the
inevitable, early result. In reality, half of all couples
who are trying to conceive do not succeed for at least
six months. Hence knowledge of this and a few other
simple facts is useful for those who have decided to try
for a baby. Biologically, women are at their most fertile
before the age of 25 but the rising number of first-time
mothers in their 30s and even 40s, shows that age is not
a critical factor. Both men and women are advised to
adopt a healthy lifestyle before they try to conceive and
there are four main aspects to this.

Firstly and most importantly, smokers should make
this the time to give up once and for all. Smoking
lowers fertility in both men and women and has proven
deleterious effects upon a developing foetus and on
a child after birth. A person who has not been able to
give up smoking for the sake of his or her own health
should give it up for the sake of the hoped-for child.

Secondly, men should reduce their consumption of alcohol to within the current safe limits of no more than 21 units per week while women are advised not to drink at all. Excess drinking has an adverse effect on a man's sperm and alcohol consumption by a woman at the time of conception may increase the risk of abnormalities in the foetus. In any event, women are now advised not to drink during pregnancy.

Thirdly, prospective mothers in particular are advised to lose excess weight before trying to conceive as this reduces the likelihood of weight-related problems arising during pregnancy or following **CHILD-BIRTH**. Losing weight can be incorporated into the adoption of a generally more healthy lifestyle by both partners, e.g. eating a good, varied, low-fat diet, taking regular exercise and getting plenty of sleep.

Fourthly, it is important as far as it is possible, to avoid undue stress when trying to conceive. Stress and worry reduce the chances of conception and failure to conceive can in itself be a source of tension.

It is obviously sensible to have sex during the woman's fertile period which lasts from about seven days before to one day after ovulation. However, it is important not to become obsessed about becoming pregnant since this can simply become a further source of anxiety. It is all too easy for a failure to conceive to place a strain upon an otherwise good relationship. Many couples find that it is only when they go beyond the stage of looking for signs of, or expecting, pregnancy every month, that they finally conceive and often this comes as a very welcome surprise.

GENETIC SCREENING AND COUNSELLING

Genetic screening and counselling is not routinely offered to all people. However, it is available to those whose family history suggests that they may be at risk of passing on a genetically determined disease to their offspring. A medical history is obtained and various tests may be carried out, for example, on samples of blood, to determine the genetic status of the person concerned. He or she can then receive counselling about the potential risks to any future children.

It is often the case that people do not know that they are carriers of a genetic disorder. This is because the genes involved may be recessive (present but masked) and the individuals concerned are well and not affected in any way by the disorder. The problem only becomes apparent when two affected individuals produce a child with a recognized genetic disorder. In this case, the couple can be counselled about the risks to any further children and can make decisions based upon the best possible medical advice. The most well-known genetic disorder for which screening is available is cystic fibrosis but there are very many others. Recent scientific advances, especially the mapping of the human genome, offer considerable hope that in the future, many severe genetic disorders can be prevented and/or successfully treated.

INFERTILITY AND ASSISTED CONCEPTION

Problems with fertility cover a broad spectrum of conditions, ranging from those which are minor and relatively simple to treat to true infertility, often affecting just one partner. Modern, sophisticated techniques of assisted conception make it possible for some couples with a significant infertility problem to have a baby. However, the route of assisted conception is frequently difficult, highly stressful, expensive and by no means always rewarded with success.

If, after one year of regular sexual intercourse throughout the woman's monthly cycle, PREGNANCY has not occurred, it is wise to seek medical advice. Initial checks and tests may be carried out by the family doctor in the first instance. The doctor may wish the woman to take her temperature on a daily basis so that the slight rise that occurs at the time of ovulation can be detected. This is one simple means of determining whether ovulation is taking place. Urine samples may be sent for laboratory analysis to check for the hormones which stimulate ovulation. If ovulation is taking place, the couple may be advised to try for a little longer, ensuring that they have intercourse during the woman's fertile period. They will probably also be advised about lifestyle factors (as described above on page 218) to increase their chances of success.

If there is still no pregnancy, further investigative tests will probably be recommended to see if there is a readily identifiable cause for the problem. Some tests may be carried out by the family doctor but the likelihood is that the couple will be referred to an infertility clinic which may involve some delay.

It is all too easy for each person to think that the problem lies with their partner, especially if either has already had children in a previous relationship. In fact, no assumptions can be made as problems affecting fertility can arise at any time, for example as a result of an infection. Studies suggest that in 30 per cent of cases, the problem lies with the woman and in a further 30 per cent, with the man and in the remainder, there are either a number of contributory factors or the cause is not identified. The latter can sometimes be the hardest to deal with while still holding out the hope that a pregnancy will eventually occur at some stage.

The three main causes of female infertility are:

1 Failure to ovulate which is the most common. There may be several reasons why the ovaries are not functioning normally including hormonal imbalance, a failure in the maturation, release or provision of eggs and structural damage to the organs themselves. Hormonal causes may respond to appropriate drug treatment.

2 A more generalized hormonal imbalance, perhaps involving pituitary gland hormones. Once again, this may be amenable to drug treatment.

3 Structural problems involving the Fallopian tubes or UTERUS. The Fallopian tubes are susceptible to damage and blockage as a result of pelvic infection and inflammation and the build-up of scar tissue. Similar damage can be caused by scar tissue and adhesions from abdominal surgery, a previous ECTOPIC PREGNANCY, or ENDOMETRIOSIS that is affecting the Fallopian tubes. Tubal blockage can be difficult to treat and is becoming increasingly common as a result of SEXUALLY TRANSMITTED DISEASES such as CHLAMYDIA. The uterus may be affected by a congenital abnormality, FIBROIDS, POLYPS, adhesions and scar tissue, all of which make it difficult for a fertilized egg to implant. This is a different problem in the sense that conception has occurred but the early embryo does not then receive the opportunity to grow. It may be possible to treat the defect in the uterus so that implantation and pregnancy can occur.

Problems with the cervical mucus are a fourth less common cause of female infertility, responsible for about 5 per cent of cases. The mucus can be too scanty or too thick to allow the passage of sperm or can even contain antibodies that attack sperm.

Diagnosis of female infertility involves a battery of techniques. These include hormone assay, ovarian function tests, ultrasound scans, endometrial biopsy by **HYSTEROSCOPY, LAPAROSCOPY** and hysterosalpinogram (HSG) – an X-ray technique requiring the injection of a dye to detect problems in the uterus and Fallopian tubes. Treatment depends upon the nature of the problem but many women who are initially infertile can be helped to conceive.

There are various causes of male infertility which include the following:

1 Anatomical problems such as damage caused by scar tissue following pelvic or prostate gland surgery which may interfere with ejaculation. Anatomical damage, including blockage of the vasa deferentia can be caused by previous pelvic infections, especially **GONORRHOEA**. (Retrograde ejaculation, where semen is forced backwards into the bladder, is a relatively common problem following surgical removal of the prostate gland. This is a cause of infertility but one which is not usually a problem since the operation is generally performed on older men.)

2 Reduced numbers of normal sperm or low sperm count which may be caused by numerous different factors. These include hormonal imbalance, genetic factors, previous injury, infection or radiotherapy

either directly or indirectly affecting the testicles, and environmental factors such as exposure to chemicals or radiation. Also, certain medical conditions such as **VARICOCELE** or **HYDROCELE** among others. Studies have shown that the number of normal sperm being produced by British men, particularly those in younger age groups, has declined dramatically. At the same time, there has been an increase in the proportion of ineffective, abnormal sperm in the samples that have been analysed. Both these factors are a cause for concern and it is thought that environmental (chemical) pollution may be one contributory cause. There may be implications for future population levels, if present trends continue.

3 Impaired efficiency in the operation of sperm. This includes sperm which are either unable to 'swim' or do so only weakly and so cannot pass through the cervical mucus. It also includes those which are able to move but lack the ability to penetrate the ovum and effect **FERTILIZATION**.

4 Problems caused by the immune system. A man may develop, in effect, an autoimmune response in which his immune system treats his sperm as 'foreign' and produces antibodies against them. This is particularly common in men who have had a **VASECTOMY**, occurring in about half of all of those who have undergone this procedure. This is an additional reason for a man to think very carefully before undergoing vasectomy. Even if surgical reversal of a vasectomy (known as vasovasostomy) is possible and seemingly successful, it may not necessarily restore fertility. It is also possible for the woman's immune system to produce antibodies against her partner's sperm, rendering them ineffective.

A whole battery of tests have been developed in recent years to try and establish the cause of a man's infertility. These include tests to count the number of sperm and to assess their fitness, survival and ability to fertilize an egg. Also, scans on the reproductive organs to see if there is a physical abnormality and blood or urine tests to check hormone levels. If the cause can be established, there is usually some form of treatment which can be attempted, commonly involving drug therapy or possibly surgery, to try and improve the situation. The success or otherwise of treatment very much depends upon the nature of the problem and it may remain unlikely that the man will be able to father a child by natural means.

However, some infertile couples can be helped to have their own child through a variety of assisted conception techniques. The most familiar of these is in-vitro fertilization (IVF) in which mature eggs are removed from a woman's ovaries and mixed in the laboratory, with sperm obtained from her husband. A maximum of three fertilized eggs or early embryos are then introduced into the woman's uterus in the hope that at least one of them will implant and produce a pregnancy. It is generally necessary for the woman to undergo treatment with hormonal drugs, which may produce side effects, in order to obtain mature eggs which must then be harvested by means of laparoscopy. Following the transfer of embryos into the womb, other hormonal preparations may be given to favour pregnancy.

There are several variations on the basic process of IVF, involving, in some cases, manipulation of the sex cells (gametes) or of the embryo itself:

• **Gamete Intrafallopian Transfer** (GIFT) involves the transplanting of sperm and eggs into the Fallopian tube in the hope that fertilization will take place naturally.

• **Zygote Intrafallopian Transfer** (ZIFT) involves the transfer of a fertilized egg/first stage embryo into the Fallopian tube.

• **Tubal Embryo Stage Transfer** (TEST) involves the transfer of embryos fertilized and grown in a laboratory into the Fallopian tube, rather than into the uterus as in classic IVF.

- **Peritoneal Ovum and Sperm Transfer** (POST) involves sperm and eggs that have been mixed together in a syringe being injected into the abdominal cavity close to the open ends of the Fallopian tubes.

All these techniques have, as their final aim, the production of a healthy pregnancy but the whole process of assisted conception can be an incredibly stressful one. For the woman, especially, there may be side effects from drug treatments and pain or discomfort from surgical procedures. The couple may well have to cope with the disappointment and psychological impact of failed treatments. Few people realize the degree of strain involved until they embark upon the process and so counselling is an essential part of any course of infertility treatment. For some couples, this will inevitably involve helping them to come to terms with the fact that treatment has failed and that it is not appropriate for them to continue.

Unfortunately, even when a couple can potentially be helped by infertility treatment, they may not be able to obtain such treatment through the National Health Service. While excellent private treatment is available from some clinics, this route may be financially out of reach for many couples. It is all too easy for a couple to use up all their savings on fertility treatment which, in the end, fails to work.

It is widely acknowledged that couples seeking or undergoing these treatments can become totally absorbed or even obsessed with their desire to have a baby, to the exclusion of almost everything else in life. This, in itself, can sometimes become a greater problem than the original childlessness. In the past, when little could be done to help, people were probably better able to accept childlessness with a passing regret and sadness. Concerns have been raised that in the modern Western world, people now expect and demand to have children as a right and infertility treatment has possibly made this view more prevalent.

Such moral arguments have certainly surrounded the other means by which some childless couples have obtained a baby – buying an infant from a Third World country or resorting to paid surrogacy.

Surrogacy involves the use of another woman to bear a child for the couple involved. Sometimes, the child is the biological offspring of the male partner and the surrogate mother but this is not always the case. Serious ethical questions are raised about the rights of a child to know its biological heritage as opposed to the rights of wealthy people to buy a baby at almost any price.

At the present time, surrogacy itself is legal in Britain but paying the woman who bears the child (other than for certain expenses) is not. There are likely to be tighter controls in the near future and the organisations that presently make surrogacy arrangements are private ones, charging large fees and mainly based abroad.

CHAPTER 14

Conception and pregnancy

CONCEPTION

Biologically speaking, conception occurs at the moment of fertilization. This takes place when the nucleus of a sperm and an egg unite to produce a unique early embryo called a zygote which has a full, individual complement of chromosomes. Fertilization takes place high up in a Fallopian tube near its corresponding ovary and the early embryo travels down the tube towards the womb, undergoing cell division as it does so. The embryo takes about three days to reach the womb where it initially moves about freely, being nourished by the secretions of cells of the ENDOMETRIUM (lining of the womb).

After one week, the embryo has become differentiated into a hollow ball of cells called a blastocyst and it is at this stage that it implants into the womb. The blastocyst becomes embedded in the endometrium which itself grows outwards to surround the embryo. Eventually, after about eight weeks, tissues from both the growing embryo and the endometrium develop to form a special organ called the placenta. This iscomposed of both maternal and embryonic tissues and it attaches the embryo to the uterus. It allows oxygen and nutrients to pass from the mother's blood to that of the embryo although maternal and foetal blood circulation remains separate. Waste products produced by the embryo pass into the maternal blood supply and are eliminated. The placenta produces hormones to regulate the pregnancy and it stores glycogen which can be converted to glucose to provide energy, if required. The placenta weights about 906 g (2 lbs) when fully developed and it is expelled soon after birth.

PREGNANCY

Gestation is a biological term for the length of time between fertilization and birth and it is often used comparatively between different mammalian species. Pregnancy is a very similar term and is strictly the period of time between the first day of a woman's last menstrual period and the delivery of a full-term child. Pregnancy lasts for approximately 40 weeks or 280 days. Whatever the biological/scientific definitions, most women would probably not consider themselves to be pregnant until their embryo is implanted in the womb. There is a great deal of sense in this viewpoint since it is known that many embryos do not implant but are 'lost' for some reason and in any event, pregnancy is not reliably detectable, even with today's more sophisticated tests, prior to implantation. Pregnancy tests usually involve the analysis of a urine (or blood) sample for the presence of the hormone, human chorionic gonadotrophin (HCG). Early physical signs of pregnancy include cessation of menstrual periods, tenderness and/or enlargement of the breasts, nausea and **MORNING SICKNESS**.

Human pregnancy is divided into three, approximately three-month periods called trimesters. During the first trimester, the embryo undergoes very rapid differentiation developing all the rudimentary major organs and the eyes and limb buds. The heart starts beating at four weeks but this cannot be detected externally until the end of the first trimester when the embryo, now called a foetus, is about 5 cm in length. The placenta develops rapidly during this period and there are huge hormonal changes in the mother which often cause nausea gravidarum or morning sickness. The main symptoms are feelings of nausea and actual vomiting which may be provoked by the sight and smell of certain foods or arise spontaneously. A drop in blood sugar is believed to be a contributory factor and the main remedy is to prevent this by eating small, carbohydrate-rich snacks at frequent intervals, especially before rising in the morning. Drinking extra fluids helps to prevent dehydration if vomiting is occurring. In severe cases, a condition called **HYPER-EMESIS GRAVIDARUM** can develop due to frequent vomiting which depletes the mother of fluid, electrolytes and vitamins. Admittance to hospital is necessary so that fluids can be given intravenously. In all but the severest cases, anti-nausea preparations are not recommended and must only be taken under medical supervision.

During the second trimester, hormone levels stabilize and to many women's relief, morning sickness usually disappears. The foetus grows rapidly and its organs and external features continue to develop so that it soon becomes recognisable as a baby. It moves around a great deal during this state and many women can detect this quite early on. By the end of the second trimester, the foetus is about 30 cm long and due to its rapid growth the uterus has expanded considerably and the mother has noticeably changed shape!

In the third trimester, the foetus continues to grow and mature and fully fills all the space in the uterus so that it can no longer move around easily. By this stage, the mother's abdomen is so distended that nearby organs are compressed and displaced to some extent. This can cause discomfort for the mother, common problems being indigestion and heartburn and urinary frequency due to pressure on the bladder. Backache is another frequent problem due to the extra weight of the pregnancy. During the last trimester, the baby usually assumes a head down position and shortly before birth the head becomes 'engaged' in the bowl of the mother's pelvis.

Pregnant women nowadays are assailed with a wealth of medical and non-medical advice which can sometimes seem bewildering and cause anxiety. In general, common sense should prevail and it is best to continue to follow a healthy lifestyle which involves eating a good and varied diet, taking regular exercise and getting plenty of sleep. Doctors generally advise avoidance of alcohol, as well as certain foods such as soft cheeses and paté, which may harbour harmful organisms, but there are few real prohibitions during pregnancy which should be a positive experience for women. Life should continue to be enjoyed in as full and normal a way as possible, although some of the discomforts of pregnancy – morning sickness, fatigue and being larger and heavier than usual – obviously interfere with this to some extent.

Good antenatal care throughout the pregnancy, during which the health of the mother and foetus are closely monitored, ensures that any potential problems are usually promptly identified. Antenatal checks involve a range of tests and procedures but most of them are simple and straightforward and soon become a matter of routine. Examples include measurement of weight and a check on blood pressure, external abdominal examination and listening to the foetal heartbeat, at least one ultrasound scan and the testing of one or more blood samples to check for immunity to rubella (German measles, which can harm a developing foetus), rhesus factor compatibility and indicators for certain congenital disorders such as Down's syndrome. All women are given folic acid supplements, as soon as their pregnancy is confirmed, to guard against the possible development of neural tube defects such as spina bifida. Folic acid has been shown to be protective and women who are planning pregnancy may also be advised to take this supplement. The techniques employed during antenatal care have become increasingly sophisticated and it is now sometimes possible to detect, for example, heart problems in an unborn child. This allows paediatricians to make the best possible decision for the baby which, in rare cases, may even involve corrective microsurgery before birth.

MISCARRIAGE

Miscarriage is the spontaneous or natural abortion of a foetus before the 28th week of pregnancy. After 28 weeks, the loss of the foetus is termed a STILLBIRTH. Miscarriage is an extremely common occurrence. It is believed that 15–20 per cent of all conceptions end in miscarriage, the vast majority occurring in the first three months of pregnancy. Many of these occur through the body's natural rejection of a foetus that is defective in some way. Other causes include defects in the **UTERUS, CERVIX** or **PLACENTA** or infections and conditions that affect them. Alternatively, other diseases and conditions present in the body may indirectly bring about a miscarriage or contribute towards it, as may exposure to certain environmental factors such as some pathogenic organisms, radiation, tobacco smoke and chemicals. The symptoms of miscarriage are bleeding and uterine cramps but if they are slight, bed rest and medical intervention may successfully ensure the continuation of the pregnancy. Sometimes a threatened miscarriage can be averted for a period of time until the foetus is more mature and more likely to survive outside the womb. Miscarriage is usually inevitable when there is severe bleeding and cramps, especially at an early stage in pregnancy. However, if the woman is carrying twins or triplets, it is not unknown for one foetus to be lost and another to be preserved.

HABITUAL MISCARRIAGE is the term used when a woman has lost a foetus at the same stage in pregnancy three or more times. Sometimes a foetus may die in the womb but fail to be expelled and this is termed a **MISSED MISCARRIAGE**. This may result in a **SEPTIC MISCARRIAGE** in which an infection arises as a result of deterioration of the foetus and placenta. Symptoms of a septic miscarriage include abdominal pain, fever and bleeding. Hospital admission is necessary so that appropriate treatment can be given.

Miscarriage may be a common occurrence but it is, nonetheless, traumatic and distressing for the couple concerned. Feelings of grief and guilt are commonly experienced and the woman needs to be reassured that the miscarriage has not occurred because of something she has or has not done. It also helps to know that most women go on to have a subsequent normal pregnancy and give birth to a healthy child. It is very natural for the woman to want to become pregnant again as soon as possible following her miscarriage. Usually, she is advised to wait for six months before trying to conceive again in order to give herself time to recover physically and emotionally from the effects of the miscarriage.

A subsequent pregnancy is often accompanied by heightened feelings of anxiety until the time of the earlier miscarriage has been passed and a woman may need a great deal of reassurance that this time, all is well. The emotional trauma is now more fully understood than was the case previously and professional help is available for women who have suffered a miscarriage. The Miscarriage Association is a national organisation that provides support. Any woman who continues to experience emotional trauma or who becomes depressed should seek professional help.

ABORTION

Abortion is surgical or medical intervention in a

pregnancy to bring about a termination before the foetus is viable. Abortion is a controversial and emotive issue which stirs up the passions both of those opposed and those in favour of the procedure. Varying degrees of regulation may be applied in those countries which permit the carrying out of abortions. In the UK, a woman is permitted to have an abortion if two doctors agree that the continuation of the pregnancy places her physical or mental health in jeopardy. It is also permitted if the foetus is deemed to be at risk of being born with physical or mental disabilities, most of which are detected by antenatal screening.

Legally, an abortion can be carried out up to 24 weeks from the date of the woman's last menstrual period but, in practice, the cut-off point is usually a great deal earlier and most abortions are performed before 12 weeks. (Twenty-four weeks is the date at which a baby is now deemed to be potentially viable.) Later abortions, generally carried out between 16 and 20 weeks' gestation, are usually performed due to serious abnormalities detected in the foetus or because a problem has arisen which directly threatens the woman's life.

Abortion is available on the NHS or can be obtained at a private clinic, as long as the legal requirements are met. A GP may refer a woman for an abortion but two charitable organisations, the British Pregnancy Advisory Service (BPAS) and the Pregnancy Advisory

Service (PAS) can be alternatively contacted for help and advice. Pre-abortion counselling, to deal with the emotional impact, as well as the physical aspects of the process, is extremely important and should be offered at some stage prior to the procedure being carried out.

Several methods of terminating a pregnancy are in use and the one which is employed is mainly governed by the stage that has been reached. Almost all early abortions (before 12 weeks gestation) are performed by a method known as **VACUUM ASPIRATION**. A light general anaesthetic is given and the cervix is then gently dilated to allow the passage of a narrow tube. An electric pump is then employed to suck out the contents of the uterus.

Induction or induced labour using an intravenous infusion of prostaglandins is commonly used for later abortions of 12 to 20 weeks. A few hours after the infusion is given, contractions in the uterus begin and labour follows to expel the foetus and placenta. The labour may be painful although it is generally less severe than that which occurs with a full-term birth. Pain relief is available and can be given as required, but the woman may be required to have a D and C, carried out under a general anaesthetic, to make sure that all the contents of the womb have been expelled.

Dilation and evacuation (D and E) is another less commonly used method of later stage abortion for pregnancies beyond 12 weeks. Prostaglandin gel is used to soften the cervix which may take up to two days to occur. The abortion is then carried out under a general anaesthetic with the cervix carefully held open with dilators and a curette and vacuum suction used to loosen and remove the contents of the womb. Both D and E and induction require a short stay in hospital (perhaps one night and one day) in order to ensure that all is well.

The one medical, as opposed to surgical, method of abortion is the so-called 'abortion pill'. It can only be used up until the 9th week of pregnancy or 63 days from the date of the last menstrual period and is not suitable for all women. The woman is required to attend a hospital or other clinic where she is given a 600 mg dose of Mifepristone™ which is an anti-progesterone preparation that acts against the progesterone necessary to sustain the pregnancy. The woman stays at the clinic for about two hours to ensure that the drug does not make her sick and then she is able to return home. Once 48 hours have elapsed, the patient returns to the clinic when a pessary containing prostaglandin is inserted into the vagina. This usually induces contractions similar to menstrual cramps and abortion/miscarriage within about six hours. If all is well, the woman is usually able to return home later in the day, but a minority of patients require a D and C which must be carried out under a general anaesthetic. The abortion pill has a success rate of 95 per cent.

There is some bleeding following an abortion, whatever the method used, which usually lasts for about two weeks but becomes increasingly light. Sanitary pads should be used and not tampons and sexual intercourse should be avoided. Any signs of infection, such as an increase in bleeding, abdominal pains or tenderness, fever, headaches or sickness should be reported to a doctor so that appropriate treatment can be given. Untreated, or unsuspected, infections such as **CHLAMYDIA** and **GONORRHOEA** can gain access to the higher reproductive organs following an abortion so vigilance is needed to safeguard future fertility. However, the risk of infection is no greater than that following childbirth or natural miscarriage, and abortion does not usually affect fertility or child-bearing.

Abortion is carried out for a variety of different reasons and the emotions that it engenders are equally complex. These may range from a feeling of profound relief that an unwanted pregnancy has been taken away, through grief, guilt, anger and depression. It is not only the woman who experiences these feelings – her partner may be equally affected if a longed-for pregnancy has had to be terminated for medical reasons. It is extremely important for these feelings to be openly acknowledged if they are not to cause problems in the future. Family and friends can help but professional therapy or counselling may be needed.

CHAPTER 15

Disorders of pregnancy

Good antenatal and obstetric care mean that serious problems relating to pregnancy and childbirth are usually promptly identified and dealt with. Maternal deaths are, fortunately, very rare but cannot be prevented altogether. There is a greater risk of death or damage to the infant if complications arise during childbirth, but this is also uncommon.

ECTOPIC PREGNANCY

An ectopic pregnancy is one which develops in an organ other than the uterus, and almost always in a Fallopian tube (in 99 per cent of cases). It usually occurs because the Fallopian tube is damaged or partially blocked, hence obstructing the normal passage of the fertilized egg down to the womb. As stated previously, Fallopian tubes can easily be damaged by previous **PELVIC INFLAMMATORY DISEASE** or **CHLAMYDIA** or **GONORRHOEA INFECTION**, with certain types of **CONTRACEPTION (IUD, PROGESTERONE-ONLY MINI-PILL)** posing additional slight risk. About one per cent of pregnancies are ectopic and the rate is slightly higher in first pregnancies.

Ectopic pregnancy is described as subacute or acute. In the subacute form, symptoms (including abdominal and referred shoulder pain, vaginal bleeding and fainting) may arise but this is not always the case. One or two menstrual periods may have been missed but a pregnancy test may not always be positive. It is believed that in many such cases, the embryo dies naturally during the first few weeks as it fails to thrive or be sustained in its abnormal situation. If this occurs, the tissue may well be naturally absorbed and dealt with by the mother's body. If the embryo continues to survive, a subacute ectopic pregnancy is usually detected between eight to ten weeks of gestation (or earlier), by which time symptoms may well be present. Ultrasound scanning and laparoscopy may be used to diagnose the condition and surgery to remove the embryo and possibly the Fallopian tube may be required. Alternatively, the embryo may be injected with a lethal substance which causes it do die and eventually be reabsorbed – a situation which hopefully preserves the Fallopian tube.

Drastic measures are necessary because, if not treated, the growing embryo eventually ruptures the Fallopian tube – the potentially fatal condition called acute ectopic pregnancy. Rupture of the tube causes severe pain, possible haemorrhage, low blood pressure and shock with symptoms of pallor, dizziness, sweating, weak, rapid pulse and irregular breathing and confusion. This is a medical emergency, requiring immediate admittance to hospital for surgical removal of the embryo and the Fallopian tube.

In extremely rare cases, the embryo may attach elsewhere in the abdominal cavity, perhaps to the ovary itself or to a portion of the bowel. The embryo or foetus invariably dies and, if its presence is diagnosed, it is surgically removed. Very rarely, if undetected, the body may react to its presence by encapsulating the foetus with scar tissue. In one recent, well-publicized case, an elderly European woman, who had suffered from abdominal pains for many years, was found to have an encapsulated foetus attached by adhesions to her digestive tract, which was thought to have been there for about 30 years!

ABRUPTIO PLACENTAE

Abruptio placentae or placental abruption is the partial or complete separation of the placenta from the uterine wall. It generally arises after the 20th week of pregnancy, although may occur earlier and the cause is unknown. It affects about 0.5 per cent of pregnancies, occurring especially in women who have already given birth to two or more children. Placental separation always results in blood loss but the severity of this depends upon the degree of separation. Slight separation may result in a light loss of blood which may only require close monitoring (by ultrasound and other external methods) and bed rest. A moderate separation describes the situation in which one quarter of the placenta becomes detached and between 500 to 1,000 mls of blood are lost. The mother requires a blood transfusion and the baby may well be delivered early by Caesarean section, especially if it has reached a viable stage. The most dangerous situation is when the separation is severe and this results in great maternal blood loss, contraction of the uterus and the potential development of shock, which may be fatal. In this emergency situation, the foetus has to be delivered immediately by Caesarean section and the mother given blood transfusions and other treatment to stop the bleeding in order to save her life. The foetus may not survive.

Occasionally, especially as the condition is developing or perhaps if the degree of separation is not initially too great, the blood loss may be retained within the uterus (concealed haemorrhage). This can also be dangerous as it may mask the severity of the condition. Abruptio placentae is one of the main causes of haemorrhage in pregnancy but, fortunately, it is relatively rare.

PLACENTA PRAEVIA

Placenta praevia is a rare condition in which the

placenta develops in the lower sector of the uterus over the cervix. This usually causes no symptoms until late in pregnancy when there is placental separation and bleeding which must be dealt with. The condition may be diagnosed by means of ultrasound scanning and, in 60 per cent of cases, the baby needs to be delivered immediately by Caesarean section. As with ABRUPTIO PLACENTAE, the risk of developing placenta praevia increases with age and number of previous deliveries, although the exact cause is unknown.

PRE-ECLAMPSIA

Pre-eclampsia is a potentially serious condition in which a pregnant woman's blood pressure rises to a high level when it had previously been stable. It is often accompanied by oedema or fluid retention, commonly noticed as puffiness and swelling in the feet, lower legs and face, etc. Admittance to hospital for bed rest, monitoring and treatment to reduce the hypertension is essential and to prevent the development of full ECLAMPSIA.

ECLAMPSIA

Eclampsia is an acute and life-threatening condition for mother and child which is fortunately rare and can usually be prevented by the treatment of the PRE-ECLAMPSIA by which it is preceded. Eclampsia usually occurs in the third trimester of pregnancy or immediately after childbirth and produces symptoms of headache, anxiety, fever, blurred vision, rapid pulse, exaggerated reflexes and decreased urinary output. Grand mal convulsions, coma, extreme hypertension and oedema are characteristic. The uterus goes into spasm, cutting off or greatly reducing the blood supply to the foetus, causing a lack of oxygen which may result in death or damage. The foetus may also be harmed by anti-convulsive drugs given to the mother but, in any event, delivery is usually effected straight away by means of Caesarean section. Delivery usually improves the situation for the mother but occasionally the convulsions can resume and may prove fatal. Delivery of the baby, anti-convulsive therapy and drug treatment to reduce hypertension and sedate the brain are all essential.

Eclampsia is more likely to develop in a first pregnancy and it is particularly associated with multiple pregnancies. A woman who has previously had the condition is at risk of developing it again in a subsequent pregnancy. There also appears to be some familial risk in that a woman whose mother was affected is more likely to develop the condition herself. About half of all cases of eclampsia occur during late stage pregnancy, one quarter during labour itself and the remainder soon after childbirth during the first twenty-four hours. The development of a **HYDATIFORM MOLE** is a further risk factor for eclampsia.

HYDATIFORM MOLE

A hydatiform mole is an abnormal development of the placenta in which the membrane known as the chorion that surrounds the embryo degenerates and is replaced by a series of fluid-filled, grape-like sacs. The embryo dies and disintegrates but the uterus enlarges and fluid and cysts are eventually discharged to the outside. Nausea and vomiting may be accompanying symptoms. The condition may be suspected if no foetal heartbeat is detected by the third month of a confirmed pregnancy.

Hydatiform mole produces unusually high levels of human chorionic gonadotrophin (HCG hormone) and so analysis of a blood sample helps to confirm the condition which may also be detected by means of ultrasound scanning. A D and C or other technique may be employed to remove the mole.

Most moles are benign but rarely, a malignant growth called choriocarcinoma can develop from a hydatiform mole. Hence a woman who has had this condition receives ongoing monitoring with periodic blood tests to check for the presence of HCG. It is usual for the woman to be advised to avoid pregnancy for one year.

HYDRAMNIOS (OR '-NION')

Hydramnios (or '-nion') describes a condition in which there is an excessive quantity of amniotic fluid surrounding the foetus, usually developing by, or beyond, the fifth month of pregnancy. The normal quantity of fluid is about one litre but in hydramnios it is double that amount. Symptoms produced include a swollen uterus (which causes breathlessness) and oedema affecting the legs and abdomen.

The fluid may collect gradually or suddenly but the cause is unknown, although the condition is particularly associated with multiple pregnancy and maternal diabetes. Hydramnios may cause a premature birth but is also associated with foetal abnormalities, particularly of the gastrointestinal tract and central nervous system. The condition is usually diagnosed by means of an ultrasound scan and the woman may require admittance to hospital for rest and monitoring.

HYPEREMESIS GRAVIDARUM

Hyperemesis gravidarum is a rare condition in which the woman develops extremely severe vomiting early in her pregnancy which depletes her of fluid and electrolytes and leads to dehydration. It is distinct from the milder MORNING SICKNESS which is commonly experienced by women during early pregnancy. Hyperemesis gravidarum requires hospital admittance so that fluids can be given intravenously, along with anti-vomiting drugs. There is a risk of liver damage in the mother and rarely, if the condition cannot be controlled, termination of the pregnancy may be the only option to safeguard the woman's health.

CHAPTER 16

Labour, childbirth and breastfeeding

Labour, birth and caring for the newborn are subjects which usually merit a book in themselves and hence will be described only briefly here. Pregnant women, especially those who are first-time mothers, receive excellent information from antenatal classes to prepare them for childbirth and caring for a newborn baby. Also, in recent years, the emphasis has been very much on giving mothers freedom of choice on how their labour will be managed and women are encouraged to make a 'birth plan' detailing their preferred options.

LABOUR AND CHILDBIRTH

In medical terms, labour is considered to have three stages although the woman herself may be unaware of the finer distinctions between them! During the first stage, uterine contractions begin and the cervix becomes dilated to its fullest extent (about 10 cm in diameter) to allow the passage of the baby's head. The amniotic membranes rupture releasing the fluid surrounding the baby to the exterior. The contractions of the uterus become more intense and frequent as the first stage of labour progresses.

The second stage lasts from full dilation of the cervix until the moment that the baby is born and is the phase when the mother actively pushes the baby down through the birth canal to the outside. Contractions of abdominal and uterine muscles aid the mother's efforts to move the baby downwards. When the baby's head appears at the vaginal opening and does not slip backwards between contractions, it is said to be 'crowning'. Eventually, the skin and tissues of the **PERINEUM** thin and stretch and may tear to allow the baby's head to pass to the outside. Sometimes a controlled cut called an episiotomy is made to allow this to occur. Once the head is delivered, the rest of the body usually follows quickly with the next contraction marking the close of the second stage of labour. The baby's nose and air passages are cleared of any adhering material and he or she is quickly handed to the mother. Once the umbilical cord has stopped pulsating, it is clamped and cut. The baby is quickly cleaned, weighed and wrapped, and an Apgar score test, which ascertains the condition of a newborn infant, is carried out.

The third stage of labour is marked by a resumption of contractions to expel the placenta. Usually, an intramuscular injection of a drug such as Syntometrine™ is given to accelerate the process (as this reduces the risk of **POSTPARTUM HAEMORRHAGE**) and this is given almost immediately after the birth of the baby. Delivery of the placenta, which is a soft organ, is normally straightforward and the woman may be almost unaware that it is taking place. The placenta is examined to make sure that it is intact and about this time, any stitches that are needed to repair a perineal tear are carried out under local anaesthetic. The uterus begins to decrease in size almost immediately once labour is over and this may be felt as tugging 'after pains' which are usually mild or uncomfortable at worst and last for only a few days.

A first labour lasts an average of 12 hours but subsequent ones are usually shorter, about eight hours. The experience of each labour is different and unique. Also, there are considerable variations in the degree of difficulty and pain experienced and labour is, and probably always will be, easier for some women than it is for others.

Occasionally, there may be a need for a doctor to directly assist in the delivery of a baby and this usually arises in the second stage of labour. Intervention may be necessary if the mother becomes exhausted as in a long labour, if the baby is large or is 'stuck' or if it becomes distressed or short of oxygen. Obstetric **FORCEPS** are specially designed to fit snugly around the baby's head without causing damage. During each contraction, the forceps are used to assist the downward passage of the baby and enable the infant to be quickly and safely delivered. **VENTOUSE DELIVERY** is another common method which uses a suction cap that is attached to the baby's head by means of a vacuum. Downward pressure is exerted during contractions to gently ease the baby out.

CAESAREAN SECTION

A Caesarean section may also be used for emergency deliveries and this involves making a small incision through the abdominal wall and into the uterus and lifting the baby out. In an emergency, the mother is more likely to be given a general anaesthetic but if the delivery is by a planned Caesarean section, epidural or spinal anaesthesia may be available.

There are a considerable number of conditions which might make a planned Caesarean section the preferred method of delivery. The operation involves making a horizontal incision low down in the abdomen to penetrate the uterus just above the cervix. (If the woman is having spinal anaesthesia, her view of the proceedings is obscured by a screen but she is kept informed at all times about what is happening.) The amniotic fluid is drawn off and then the baby is gently lifted out of the uterus, its nose and mouth are cleared and the umbilical cord is cut in the normal way. The baby can quickly be checked and given to the mother while the placenta is being removed and the uterine and abdominal walls are being stitched up.

A horizontal incision is the preferred option as it minimizes blood loss, heals well and reduces the risk of postoperative infection. The risk of the uterine scar opening during a subsequent pregnancy or normal delivery is considered to be small. Occasionally, a vertical incision has to be made – sometimes if the baby is lying in an unusual position – but this is uncommon. As with any operation, the woman needs time to recover and a longer stay in hospital than is the case with vaginal delivery may be expected. **BREAST-FEEDING** and caring for the baby may be more difficult following a Caesarean, but the problems are well understood and a woman should expect to receive sympathetic help, support and encouragement from hospital staff.

A Caesarean section is beneficial for the baby in that it is spared the trauma of the birth process. It is not squeezed out through the birth canal and so it does not have the squashed appearance or moulded head that can be the initial lot of a baby delivered vaginally! A Caesarean baby has a rounded head and smooth facial features but often needs more time to adjust to being in the outside world because of its sudden exit from the uterus. The journey through the birth canal helps to clear any amniotic fluid from the baby's lungs and stimulates the blood circulation. Hence some experts believe that gentle massage may be beneficial for a Caesarean newborn, although handling and holding the baby also helps it to adjust.

ABNORMAL PRESENTATION

Abnormal presentation is the term given to any birth in which a part of the body other than the crown of the baby's head 'presents' first at the vaginal opening. Often, but not always, doctors are aware of the situation and may have tried previously to turn the baby to a normal position by external manipulation. A breech position is the most common type of abnormal presentation and describes the situation where the baby's buttocks (or possibly a foot or feet) are the presenting part. Breech babies must be delivered in hospital and the birth may be more difficult because the head, which is the largest part of the body, is delivered last. If problems arise, assisted delivery of the head may be needed, especially if there is a risk of the baby trying to breathe before it is fully born. In other cases, a planned Caesarean section may be considered to be safer than vaginal delivery to safeguard the child.

POSTPARTUM HAEMORRHAGE

Postpartum haemorrhage is heavy bleeding following childbirth which can arise suddenly and, if severe, may be life-threatening and require emergency treatment.

Quite often, the bleeding is somewhat less severe and arises because placental tissue is retained within the uterus instead of it all being expelled as the afterbirth. Usually, a **D AND C** is carried out to remove the tissue and the woman may well need blood transfusions and subsequent iron supplements to prevent anaemia.

PREMATURE BIRTH

A premature baby is one that is born before 37 weeks of gestation, but it may sometimes only be classified as such if it weighs less than 2.5 kg or 5 lbs 8oz. Most premature babies require special supportive, intensive care, often in an incubator and the earlier the birth the greater the number of problems there are likely to be. A premature birth obviously places the parents under a great deal of strain, made worse if the baby's survival is in doubt. Hospital premature baby units make every effort to help and support parents and enable them to spend as much time with their baby as possible. It is recognized that this is vital to the wellbeing both of the infant and the parents and everything possible is done to ease what is undoubtedly a stressful time.

THE STILLBORN BABY

Sometimes, in spite of all possible precautions, something may go wrong or for reasons that remain unclear, a baby is stillborn. A stillborn child is one that is born after 28 weeks gestation showing no evidence of life. The loss of any child is recognized by most people to be one of the hardest forms of bereavement to cope with and it is all the more agonizing when it involves a baby whose birth has been longed for and anticipated. Fortunately, hospital staff and those involved with bereavement counselling recognize the enormity of this type of loss. Most hospitals encourage the parents to spend time with the baby and give it a name, to take photographs and to eventually hold a funeral service. All these measures are helpful for future healing and for coming to terms with the loss. Relatives and friends of people who have been bereaved often find it difficult to talk about the person who has died and try to avoid the subject, particularly if it involves a child. However, the best advice for those involved is to be a good listener and to allow the bereaved parents and family to talk about their loss as well as offering any practical help and support that may be needed.

THE BABY BLUES

Following childbirth, many women find themselves on an 'emotional rollercoaster', experiencing mood swings which vary from great happiness and elation to tearfulness. This syndrome, sometimes popularly called 'the baby blues' is a natural and common experience. It is probably triggered by the huge hormonal changes that occur before and after birth but, also, the woman has gone through one of human life's most significant events and so emotion is to be expected!

Most women find that these feelings pass quite quickly, especially once they have returned home and settled into their own routine. However, a few women go on to develop **POSTNATAL DEPRESSION** which can be mild or severe and usually occurs within six months of the baby's birth.

There are many symptoms which may arise but common among them are insomnia and wakefulness, even when not attending to the baby, feelings of guilt, hopelessness and inadequacy, extreme fatigue and lack of interest in life, excessive anxiety about the baby, panic feelings, thoughts about death and other morbid preoccupations, lack of concentration, tearfulness and general misery.

Anyone experiencing these symptoms needs prompt and sympathetic help and the family doctor must be consulted. Quite often, the provision of extra support and encouraging the mother to begin to do even simple, small things to build up her self-esteem may be enough to put her on the road to recovery. Sometimes drug treatment may help but caution is needed if the woman is **BREASTFEEDING**. Above all, the woman needs reassurance that she can and will recover, although this may take some time. Sadly, postnatal depression can spoil the mother's enjoyment of her baby in the first few months but there is rarely any long-term damage to their relationship.

BREASTFEEDING AND ASSOCIATED PROBLEMS

It is recognized that breastfeeding is the best option for a baby, providing it with all the necessary nutrients for the first few months of life as well as antibodies to protect against infection. Studies suggest that the benefits of breastfeeding continue into adult life, lessening later risks of obesity and heart disease, while the woman receives some protection from the possible later development of breast cancer. Breastfeeding also helps the uterus to return to its normal size, uses up excess fat laid down during pregnancy and provides some protection against pregnancy, although this should not be relied on for **CONTRACEPTION**. In spite of the fact that breastfeeding is self-evidently a natural process, it is not one that comes easily and naturally to all women. Perseverance and determination may well be needed, especially at the beginning, until the process is established. Equally, women who attempt to breastfeed but find that they are unable to continue should not worry but accept that bottle-fed babies thrive extremely well!

In the first two or three days after birth, the breasts produce a protein-rich fluid containing antibodies called colostrum, which is also a natural laxative and helps to stimulate the baby's digestion. It is well worth trying to breastfeed the baby during this time for the natural immunity that is passed on. Unfortunately, this initial stage can be a difficult one as the mother is likely to still be very tired after giving birth and some hungry babies are dissatisfied with colostrum alone. Midwives usually advise avoiding too much suckling at this stage to prevent breast soreness, but the baby may have other ideas!

The situation usually improves once milk production starts, generally by the third day. The opposite problem may now arise and many women find that they initially have too much milk, leading to **BREAST ENGORGEMENT**. The breasts become hard and uncomfortable but the problem is eased by expressing the milk and by feeding the baby. The baby may find it difficult to latch on to an engorged breast but this is seldom a problem for long. Usually, milk production quickly adjusts to the level needed to feed the baby and it is worth persevering with breastfeeding for one or two weeks until this adjustment has taken place. In order to establish breastfeeding, it may be best for the woman to concentrate on just looking after herself and the baby, relaxing and getting as much sleep as possible and keeping life as simple as circumstances allow.

The most common problems associated with breastfeeding are sore or cracked nipples during the early days, which can be very painful Restricting the time that the infant is allowed to suckle and using a device called a breast shield, along with applying protective cream or ointment are measures which should help. A crack can allow access for infection, the most common form being **MASTITIS,** with symptoms of inflammation, tenderness, fever and pain. This is treated with warm compresses and a course of antibiotics and is usually quickly resolved. Prompt treatment should avoid the development of a **BREAST ABSCESS** which may require drainage of the affected area along with antibiotic treatment. A **BLOCKED MILK DUCT** can cause the development of a localized firm lump but the blockage usually clears with feeding or massage of the affected area. A woman who is breastfeeding should be meticulous about taking care of her nipples and breasts with careful washing and drying and application of protective cream. Usually, any problems are short-lived and breastfeeding becomes easier as time goes on and the baby becomes older.

CHAPTER 17

Menopause

FEMALE MENOPAUSE OR CLIMACTERIC

The menopause is the phase in a woman's life in which the ovaries no longer release an egg cell every month and menstruation ceases. This may happen suddenly but more usually it is a gradual process, arising and proceeding between the ages of 45 and 55. The woman is normally no longer able to conceive (although CONTRACEPTION must continue to be used until the menopause is completed) and she is termed postmenopausal when periods have ceased for one year.

There is a hormonal imbalance involving the sex hormones during the menopause which may produce a range of physical symptoms that can be quite unpleasant. These include hot flushes and profuse sweating, palpitations, mood swings, lack of concentration, depression, LOSS OF LIBIDO, vaginal dryness and sleep problems.

Some women experience these symptoms quite severely while others are relatively untroubled by them. The decline and fall in oestrogen level causes gradual osteoporosis (bone loss) in postmenopausal women which increases the risk of fractures in older age.

HORMONE REPLACEMENT THERAPY (HRT)

Both menopausal symptoms and osteoporosis are helped by taking hormone replacement therapy (HRT) which involves reintroducing the sex hormones in tablet or some other form. Most doctors believe that the benefits of this in terms of protecting the bones far outweigh any potential risks and so many advocate its use.

There are, however, some dissenting views and this remains a matter of choice for each individual woman. Taking HRT produces a slight increase in the risk of developing breast cancer but it is thought to protect against heart disease and stroke, both of which pose a greater threat to postmenopausal women.

HRT is not suitable for every woman and the existence of some medical conditions, such as breast cancer, rules out its use and, as with the contraceptive pill, it can take some time to find a preparation that is best suited to each individual. One of the disadvantages used to be that most HRT preparations produced a light, monthly bleed in a woman who would normally have stopped menstruating but HRT preparations now exist for the older woman where no monthly bleed is experienced.

MALE MENOPAUSE OR 'MID-LIFE CRISIS'

In middle age, a significant number of men experience a range of ill-defined symptoms such as fatigue, loss of concentration, forgetfulness and sleep disturbances which are commonly suffered by menopausal women. In women, the symptoms are caused by a great reduction in the female hormone oestrogen which can in many instances be alleviated by hormone replacement therapy. In most men, there is only a slight reduction in the level of testosterone produced and this does not occur until older age. Hence many medical experts believe that male symptoms are not hormonally driven but caused by stress and psychological problems.

However, many men also notice a reduction in their libido or experience minor problems relating to sexual performance which may contribute to their symptoms. Some experimental studies have shown that given testosterone replacement therapy a number of men have noticed an improvement in these symptoms. Hence some doctors believe that although there is no reduction in the levels of testosterone, the hormone works less effectively in middle-aged men and this is the factor responsible for male menopausal symptoms.

Testosterone replacement therapy is a controversial treatment that is only available privately. There are concerns that giving additional testosterone to essentially healthy men may have detrimental effects, particularly an increased risk of cancer of the prostate gland. A man who is suffering from symptoms associated with a mid-life crisis should nevertheless visit his doctor for a health check-up to make sure there is nothing physically wrong. The doctor may recommend measures to deal with stress.

CHAPTER 18

Sexual orientation

HOMOSEXUALITY AND LESBIANISM

As far as is known, throughout human history and in every race and culture, there have always been people who can only find sexual fulfilment with those of their own gender. It is probably also true that in most cases homosexual men and lesbian women have always faced prejudice and hostility and that this continues to the present day.

Because they practise anal sex, homosexual men face particular risks of infection with **SEXUALLY TRANSMITTED DISEASES** and they should be careful to always practise **SAFE SEX**. Even in the more liberal, social climate that prevails today, homosexual men and lesbian women continue to experience prejudice, intolerance, discrimination or even outright hatred, and they are frequently on the receiving end of hurtful remarks or jokes or subject to physical assaults. Hence it is not surprising that many have found it hard to admit and accept their sexual orientation. Because of the stigma associated with homosexuality, many have denied their sexuality, married and had children in order to try and 'fit in', only to find that the strain of trying to be someone that they are not has led to despair, depression or breakdown.

It is recognized that it is far better for homosexual and lesbian people to accept their sexual orientation and to tell others, especially their family and close friends. Family members, especially parents, may initially find the news difficult to accept, but often this is short-lived and it is a relief to have matters out in the open. Most people quickly realize that the person whom they love is the same, whatever his or her sexual orientation, and they want that person to be happy and fulfilled. Fortunately, a strong and well-organized network of groups exist to help and support 'gay' people to overcome any problems that they may face. Parenthood is one area which is often difficult for gay couples and one which poses practical problems as well as attracting prejudice.

BISEXUALISM

Bisexual people are equally attracted to people of either sex and engage in both heterosexual and homosexual activity.

TRANSEXUALISM

Transexualism is an unusual condition in which the person is convinced that he or she has been born a member of the wrong sex. The person firmly believes that his or her biological gender is incorrect and becomes aware of this quite early in childhood. The child commonly feels that he or she is being dressed in the wrong clothes, given the wrong toys, and is unhappy about engaging in the activities enjoyed by same-sex contemporaries. The child is always happier when allowed to behave and play in a manner more appropriate to a child of the opposite sex. The condition may arise because the parents consciously or subconsciously wanted a baby of the opposite sex and unknowingly communicate this to the child. If the condition is identified in childhood, psychotherapy may help the child to accept his or her biological gender but this is not always successful.

Most transexuals are males and if they are not successfully treated in childhood, they usually become increasingly unhappy as they enter adolescence and adult life. Dressing and passing as a woman may satisfy a transsexual man for a time but he usually loathes his body to such a great extent that he eventually seeks medical and surgical treatment. Such treatment is physically and emotionally demanding and from a strictly medical point of view injurious to health, involving the taking of female hormones and disfiguring surgery. Hence it is not easy to obtain such treatment and in order to be accepted, the man will have had to have been passing himself off as a female for at least two years. Even then, treatment will not be given without prior extensive therapy and counselling. Surgery involves the removal of the male, external genital organs and the creation of an artificial vagina out of existing skin and tissue. Female hormones are given to stimulate the growth of breasts and to create a womanly shape but these may pose subsequent health risks. More than one operation may be needed along with voice and other training to achieve feminine mannerisms and behaviour. If the treatment is successful, the person may finally feel at peace although many transsexuals continue to find it impossible to form intimate or close relationships and are, of course, infertile.

CHAPTER 19

Conclusion

It can be seen that sexual and reproductive health covers many factors of human experience, extending throughout a person's lifetime. In Britain today, great emphasis is placed upon taking personal responsibility for one's own health and upon 'self-help' measures. There is no doubt that each individual has choices that he or she must make with regard to sexual and reproductive health. However, for most people at some stage in life, some aspect passes beyond individual control and medical or other help is needed. Also, education in youth, and remaining aware and informed in adult life, about developments affecting sexual and reproductive health, is invaluable. Since this subject is almost inexhaustive, some aspects may only have been slightly touched upon or possibly missed out altogether, however, it is hoped that this book will provide a useful overview for those who are interested in their sexual and reproductive health.

Glossary

abortion the removal of an embryo or foetus from the uterus, either by natural expulsion or by human intervention, before it is considered to be viable.

abruptio placentae bleeding from the placenta after the 28th week of pregnancy, which may result in the placenta becoming completely or partially detached from the wall of the uterus.

afterbirth a mass of tissue that consists of the placenta, umbilical cord and membranes, detached and expelled from the womb (uterus) during the third stage of labour following a birth.

AIDS the acronym for Acquired Immune Deficiency Syndrome caused by the human immunodeficiency virus, known as HIV, a ribonucleic acid (RNA) retrovirus.

amenorrhoea an absence of menstruation, which is normal before puberty, during pregnancy and while breast-feeding is being carried out, and following the menopause.

amniocentesis a procedure carried out to sample the amniotic fluid surrounding a foetus. It is usually carried out between the 16th and 20th week of pregnancy if a foetal abnormality is suspected.

amniotic fluid the liquid in the amniotic cavity, which is clear and composed mainly of water containing foetal cells, lipids and urine from the foetus. The amniotic fluid ('waters') is released when the membranes rupture during labour.

androgen one of a group of hormones that is responsible for the development of the sex organs and also the secondary sexual characteristics in the male. Androgens are steroid hormones, and the best-known example is testosterone. They are mainly secreted by the testes in the male but are also produced by the adrenal cortex and by the ovaries of females in small amounts.

antenatal before birth. Pregnant women attend antenatal clinics, which monitor the health of both mothers and their unborn babies.

apgar score a method of assessing the health of an infant immediately after birth, carried out at one minute and five minutes after delivery.

areola (*pl* **areolae**) the brown-coloured, pigmented ring around the nipple of the breast.

artificial insemination semen collected from a donor is inserted by means of an instrument into the vagina of a woman in the hope that she will conceive. The semen may be from her husband or partner (AIH) or from an anonymous donor (AID) and is introduced near the time of ovulation. Usually AIH is used where the partner is impotent and AID when he is sterile.

benign a term used most frequently to refer to tumours, meaning not harmful, the opposite of malignant.

birthmark *or* **naevus** an agglomeration of dilated blood vessels that creates a malformation of the skin and is present at birth. It may occur as a large port-wine stain, which can now be treated by laser, or a strawberry mark, which commonly fades in early life.

bonding the creation of a link between an infant and its parents, particularly the mother. Factors such as eye to eye contact, soothing noises, etc, are part of the process.

breast the mammary gland that produces milk. Each breast has a number of compartments with lobules surrounded by fatty tissue and muscle fibres. Milk formed in the lobules gathers in branching tubes or ducts that together form lactiferous ducts. Near the nipple the ducts form ampullae (small 'reservoirs') from which the ducts discharge through the nipple.

breast cancer a carcinoma or sarcoma, which is the commonest cancer in women.

breast screening procedures adopted to detect breast cancer as early as possible. In addition to self-examination, there are many formal programmes of screening.

breech presentation the position of a baby in the uterus whereby it would be delivered buttocks first instead of the usual head-first delivery. The baby, and possibly the mother, may be at risk in such cases.

Caesarean section a surgical operation to deliver a baby by means of an incision through the abdomen and uterus. It is performed when there is a risk to the health of the baby or mother in normal delivery, both as a planned and as an emergency procedure.

cervical a term meaning relating to the neck and often used in connection with the cervix, the neck of the womb (uterus).

cervical cancer cancer of the neck or cervix of the womb. In the precancerous stage, readily detectable changes occur in the cells lining the surface of the cervix.

cervical smear a simple test, involving scraping off some cells from the cervix and examining them microscopically. The test is carried out every three years to detect early indications of cancer and is a form of preventive medicine.

chorionic gonadotrophic hormone *or* **human chorionic gonadotrophin** (**HCG**) a hormone produced during pregnancy by the placenta, large amounts of which are present in the urine of a pregnant woman. The presence of this hormone is the basis of most pregnancy tests. It is given by injection to treat cases of delayed puberty and, with another hormone, called follicle-stimulating hormone, to women who are sterile because of a failure in ovulation. It may also be used to treat premenstrual tension.

chromosomes the rod-like structures, present in the nucleus of every body cell, that carry the genetic information or genes. Each human body cell contains 23 pairs of chromosomes, apart from the sperm and ova, half derived from the mother and half from the father. Each chromosome consists of a coiled double filament (double helix) of DNA, with genes carrying the genetic information arranged linearly along its length. The genes determine all the characteristics of each individual. Of the pairs of chromosomes, 22 are the same in males and females. The 23rd pair are the sex chromosomes, and males have one X-chromsome and one Y-chromsome, whereas females have two X-chromosomes.

circumcision a surgical removal of the foreskin (or prepuce) of the penis in males and part or all of the external genitalia (clitoris, labia minora, labia majora) in females. Female circumcision is damaging and not beneficial to a woman's health.

clitoris a small organ present in females, situated where the labial folds meet below the pubic bone. It contains erectile tissue that enlarges and hardens with sexual stimulation.

colostrum the first fluid produced by the mammary glands. It is a fairly clear fluid containing antibodies, serum and white blood cells and is produced during the first two or three days prior to the production of milk.

contraception prevention of conception.

dilatation and curettage (**D and C**) the technique whereby the cervix is opened using dilators and then the lining of the uterus is scraped using a curette. Such sampling is performed for the removal of incomplete abortions and tumours, to diagnose disease of the uterus or to correct bleeding, etc.

eclampsia convulsions that occur during pregnancy, usually at the later stages or during delivery. Although the cause is not known, the start of convulsions may be associated with cerebral oedema or a sudden rise in blood pressure. The condition requires immediate treatment as it threatens both mother and baby. Treatment is by drugs and reduction of outside stimuli, and a Caesarean section is needed.

ectopic pregnancy a pregnancy in which the fertilized egg implants outside the uterus.

ejaculation the emission of semen from the penis via the urethra. It is a reflex action produced during copulation or masturbation, and the sensation associated with it is orgasm.

embryo the first stage of development of a foetus after the fertilized ovum is implanted in the uterus until the second month.

embryo transfer the fertilization of an ovum by sperm and its development into an early embryo, outside the mother, and its subsequent implantation in the mother's uterus. Such procedures result in what is popularly termed a 'test-tube baby'.

endometriosis the occurrence of endometrium in other parts of the body, e.g. within the muscle of the uterus, in the ovary, Fallopian tubes, peritoneum and possibly the bowel. Because of the nature of the tissue, it acts in a way similar to that of the uterus lining and causes pelvic pain, bleeding and painful menstruation.

endometritis inflammation of the endometrium caused commonly by bacteria but can also be because of a virus, parasite or foreign body. It is associated with fever and abdominal pain and occurs mainly after abortion or childbirth or in women with an intrauterine contraceptive device.

endometrium the womb's mucous membrane lining that changes in structure during the menstrual cycle, becoming thicker with an increased blood supply later in the cycle. This is in readiness for receiving an embryo, but if this does not happen, the endometrium breaks down and most is lost in menstruation.

episiotomy the process of making an incision in the perineum to enlarge a woman's vaginal opening to facilitate delivery of a child. The technique is used to prevent tearing of the perineum.

erection the condition in which erectile tissue in the penis (and to some degree in the clitoris) is engorged with blood, making it swell and become hard. It is the result primarily of sexual arousal, although it can occur during sleep because of physical stimulation. It also occurs in young boys. It is a prerequisite of vaginal penetration for emission of semen.

Fallopian tubes a pair of tubes, one of which leads from each ovary to the uterus.

fertilization the fusion of sperm and ovum to form a zygote, which then undergoes cell division to become an embryo. Fertilization in humans takes place high up in the Fallopian tube near the ovary, and the fertilized egg travels down and becomes implanted in the uterus.

fibroid a type of benign tumour found in the uterus, composed of fibrous and muscular tissue and varying in size from 1 or 2 mm to a mass weighing several kilograms.

foetus *or* **fetus** an unborn child after the eighth week of development.

foreskin the prepuce, which is a fold of skin growing over the end (glans) of the penis.

gamete a mature germ or sexual cell, male or female, that can participate in fertilization, e.g. ovum and sperm.

genetic counselling the provision of advice to families about the nature and likelihood of inherited disorders and the options available in terms of prevention and management. With modern techniques of antenatal diagnosis, it is possible to determine at an early stage of a pregnancy whether a child will be abnormal.

genetic screening the procedure whereby individuals are tested to determine whether their gene make-up suggests they carry a particular disease or condition. If it is shown that someone carries a genetically linked disease, then decisions can be taken regarding future children.

genital the term used to describe anything relating to reproduction or the organs of the reproductive system.

genitalia the male or female organs of the reproductive system, often referring to the external parts only.

genital warts solid, benign growths present on the genitalia, externally or internally, which are caused by a VIRUS, the human papilloma virus (HPV). They are transmitted sexually and there is an established link between infection with certain strains of HPV and the occurrence of precancerous changes in the cervix and cervical cancer in women. Genital warts can be dealt with in several ways, e.g. cryosurgery (freezing), laser treatment and electrocautery.

genito-urinary medicine the subdiscipline concerned with all aspects of sexually transmitted diseases.

genito-urinary tract the genital and urinary organs and associated structures: kidneys, ureter, bladder, urethra and genitalia.

gestation the length of time from fertilization of the ovum to birth

gleet a discharge symptomatic of chronic gonorrhoea.

gonadotrophins *or* **gonadotrophic hormone** hormones secreted by the anterior pituitary gland. Follicle-stimulating hormone (FSH) is produced by males and females, as is luteinizing hormone, LH, (interstitial cell-stimulating hormone, ICSH) in males. FSH controls, directly or indirectly, growth of the ova and sperm, while LH/ICSH stimulates reproductive activity in the gonads.

gonads the reproductive organs that produce the gametes and some hormones. In the male and female, the gonads are the testicles and ovaries respectively.

gonorrhoea the most common venereal disease, which is spread primarily by sexual intercourse but may also be contracted through contact with infected discharge on clothing, towels, sheets etc. The causative agent is the bacterium *Neisseria gonorrhoeae*, and it affects the mucous membrane of the vagina or, in the male, the urethra.

gynaecology the subdiscipline of medicine that deals with diseases of women, particularly concerning sexual and reproductive function and diseases of reproductive organs.

hepatitis inflammation of the liver as a result of the presence of toxic substances or infection caused by viruses. The so-called hepatic viruses are designated A, B, C, D, and E. Hepatitis A and hepatitis E act in a similar way, and both produce symptoms of fever, sickness and jaundice. Serum hepatitis is caused by viruses B, C and D, the route of infection being blood or blood products. Serum hepatitis is most common where infected needles have been used among drug addicts. The infection may also be passed on by tattooing needles and also through sexual intercourse with an infected individual. All these viruses may persist in the blood for a long time and if B is involved, the condition is known as chronic type B hepatitis.

herpes infectious inflammation of the skin and mucous membranes, characterized by the development of small blisters and caused by a number of different herpes viruses. The herpes simplex virus, types I and II, are the cause of cold sores, which usually affect the lips, mouth and face. Herpes simplex is also the cause of genital herpes, in which the blisters affect the genital region.

HIV the human immunodeficiency virus responsible for the condition known as AIDS. The virus affects and destroys a group of lymphocytes (T-lymphocytes), which are part of the body's natural defences (the immune system). HIV is found in blood, other body body fluids, semen and cervical secretions and is mainy transmitted by sexual activity.

hormone a chemical substance that is naturally produced by the body and acts as a messenger. A hormone is produced by cells or glands in one part of the body and passes into the bloodstream. When it reaches another specific site, its 'target organ', it causes a reaction there, modifying the structure or function of cells, perhaps by causing the release of another hormone. Hormones are secreted by the endocrine glands, and examples are the sex hormones, e.g. testosterone, secreted by the testes, and oestradiol and progesterone, secreted by the ovaries.

hymen a thin membrane that covers the lower end of the vagina at birth and usually tears to some extent before a girl reaches puberty.

hyperemesis vomiting to excess. Hyperemesis gravidarum is excessive vomiting during pregnancy, which often begins as an exaggerated form of morning sickness. Medical intervention is imperative in this condition.

hysterectomy the surgical removal of the uterus, either by means of an abdominal incision or through the vagina. It is commonly carried out if fibroids are present or if the uterus is cancerous, and also if there is excessive bleeding.

impotence the condition when a man is unable to have sexual intercourse because of lack of penile erection or, less commonly, to ejaculate having gained an erection. The cause may be organic and the result of a condition or disease (diabetes, endocrine gland disorder) or, more commonly, psychogenic, i.e. caused by psychological or emotional problems such as anxiety, fear or guilt.

induction the commencement of labour by artificial means, either by administering drugs to produce uterine contractions or by amniotomy.

infertility the condition in which a person is unable to produce offspring naturally. Female infertility may be because of irregular or absence of ovulation, blocked Fallopian tubes, endometriosis; while a low sperm count or other deficiency in the spermatozoa can lead to male infertility. Treatment can include drug therapy, surgery or, more recently, the technique of in vitro fertilization.

insemination the introduction of semen into the vagina, whether by sexual intercourse or artificial means.

intrauterine device (**IUD**) a plastic or metal contraceptive device, often in the shape of a coil about 25 mm long, that is placed in the uterus. The device probably prevents conception by preventing potential implantation of the embryo. There are sometimes side effects, e.g. back pain and heavy menstrual bleeding, but it is a reasonably effective method.

in vitro fertilization (**IVF**) the process of fertilizing an ovum outside the body. The technique is used when a woman has blocked Fallopian tubes or when there is some other reason for sperm and ovum not uniting. The woman produces several ova (because of hormone therapy treatment), which are removed by laparoscopy, and these are mixed with sperm and incubated in culture medium until they are fertilized. At the blastocyst stage some are implanted in the mother's uterus. The first successful live birth using this technique was in 1978, when the phrase 'test-tube baby' was coined.

Kaposi's sarcoma a condition involving malignant skin tumours that form from the blood vessels. Purple lumps, as a result of the tumours, form on the feet and ankles, spreading to arms and hands. The disease is common in Africa but less so in Western countries, although it is associated with AIDS.

labia (*sing* **labium**) lips or something resembling lips, as in the folds of skin enclosing the vulva (the labia majora and minora).

labour the process of giving birth, from dilatation of the cervix to expulsion of the afterbirth. It usually commences naturally, although some labours are induced. On average, labour lasts 12 hours (less for subsequent pregnancies).

lactation the process of milk secretion by the mammary glands in the breast, which begins at the end of pregnancy. Colostrum is produced and secreted before the milk. Lactation is controlled by hormones and stops when the baby ceases to be breast fed.

lanugo a fine, downy hair. It covers the foetus between the fifth and ninth months and is lost in the ninth month so is seen only on babies born prematurely. It is also a symptom of severe anorexia nervosa.

leucorrhoea a discharge of white or yellow-coloured mucus from the vagina. It may be a normal condition, increasing before and after menstruation, but a large discharge probably indicates an infection somewhere in the genital tract. A common cause is the infection called thrush but it may also be a result of gonorrhoea, in which case the treatment will differ.

libido the sexual drive, often associated with psychiatric illnesses. Lack of libido may be the result of illness or a lack of sex hormones because of an endocrine disorder.

lightening a sensation experienced by many pregnant women, normally towards the last month of the pregnancy, when the foetus settles lower in the pelvis. This lessens the pressure on the diaphragm and breathing becomes easier.

mammary gland a gland present in the female breast that produces milk after childbirth.

mammography a special X-ray technique used to determine the structure of the breast. It is useful in the early detection of tumours and in distinguishing between benign and malignant tumours.

mammoplasty plastic surgery of the breasts to decrease or increase size and alter shape.

mastalgia pain in the breast.

mastectomy surgical removal of the breast, usually performed because of the presence of a tumour. Mastectomy may be simple, leaving the skin (and possibly the nipple) so that an artificial breast (prosthesis) can be inserted. Or it may be radical, in which case the whole breast, the pectoral muscles and the lymph nodes beneath the armpit are all removed, generally performed because a cancer has spread.

mastitis inflammation of the breast, usually caused by bacterial infection during breast-feeding, the organisms responsible gaining access through cracked nipples. Cystic mastitis does not involve inflammation, but the presence of cysts (thought to be caused by hormonal factors) causes the breast(s) to be lumpy.

menopause or **climacteric** the time in a woman's life when the ovaries no longer release an egg cell every month and menstruation ceases. The woman is normally no longer able to bear a child and the age at which the menopause occurs is usually between 45 and 55. The menopause may be marked by a gradual decline in menstruation or in its frequency, or it may cease abruptly. There is a disturbance in the balance of sex hormones, and this causes a number of physical symptoms, including palpitations, hot flushes, sweats, vaginal dryness, loss of libido and depression. In the long term, there is a gradual loss of bone (osteoporosis) in postmenopausal women, which leads to greater risk of fractures, especially of the femur in the elderly. All these symptoms are relieved by hormone replacement therapy (HRT), involving oestrogen and progesterone, which is now generally recognized to be of great benefit.

menstrual cycle and **menstruation** the cyclical nature of the reproductive life of a sexually mature female. One ovum develops and matures within a Graafian follicle in one of the ovaries. When mature, the follicle ruptures to release the egg, which passes down the Fallopian tube to the uterus. The ruptured follicle becomes a temporary endocrine gland, called the corpus luteum which secretes the hormone progesterone. Under the influence of progesterone, the uterus wall (endometrium) thickens and its blood supply increases in readiness for the implantation of a fertilized egg. If the egg is not fertilized and there is no pregnancy, the thickened endometrium is shed along with a flow of blood through the vagina (menstruation). The usual age at which menstruation starts is 12 to 15 but it can be as early as 10 or as late as 20. The duration varies and can be anything from 2 to 8 days, the whole cycle usually occupying about 29 to 30 days.

morning sickness vomiting and nausea, most common during the first three months of pregnancy.

neonatal a term meaning 'relating to the first 28 days of life'.

obstetrics the subdiscipline of medicine that deals with pregnancy and childbirth and the period immediately after birth

oestradiol the major female sex hormone. It is produced by the OVARY and is responsible for development of the breasts, sexual characteristics and premenstrual uterine changes.

oestrogen one of a group of steroid hormones secreted mainly by the ovaries and, to a lesser extent, by the adrenal cortex and placenta. (The testicles also produce small amounts.) Oestrogens control the female secondary sexual characteristics, i.e. enlargement of the breasts, change in the profile of the pelvic girdle, pubic hair growth and deposition of body fat. High levels are produced at ovulation and, with progesterone, they regulate the female reproductive cycle. Naturally occurring oestrogens include oestradiol, oestriol and oestrone. Synthetic varieties are used in the contraceptive pill and to treat gynaecological disorders.

orchidectomy removal of one or both testicles (castration), usually to treat a malignant growth.

orchidopexy the operation performed to bring an undescended testicle into the scrotum. It is undertaken well before puberty to ensure subsequent normal development.

orgasm the climax of sexual arousal which, in men, coincides with ejaculation and comprises a series of involuntary muscle contractions. In women, there are irregular contractions of the vaginal walls.

osteoporosis a loss of bone tissue because of its being resorbed, resulting in bones that become brittle and likely to fracture. It is common in menopausal women and can also be a result of long-term steroid therapy. Hormone replacement therapy is a treatment available to women.

ovarian cyst a sac filled with fluid that develops in the ovary. Most are benign but their size may cause swelling and pressure on other organs. For those cysts that do become malignant, it is possible that its discovery comes too late to allow successful treatment. Ultrasound scanning can be adopted to detect tumours at an early stage.

ovariotomy literally cutting into an ovary, but more generally used for surgical removal of an ovary or an ovarian tumour.

ovary the reproductive organ of females, which produces eggs (ova) and hormones (mainly oestrogen and progesterone). There are two ovaries, each the size of an almond, on either side of the uterus, and each contains numerous Graafian follicles in which the eggs develop. At ovulation an egg is released from a follicle. The follicles secrete oestrogen and progesterone, which regulate the menstrual cycle and the uterus during pregnancy.

ovulation the release of an egg from an ovary (i.e. from a mature Graafian follicle), which then moves down the Fallopian tube to the uterus. Ovulation is brought about by secretion of luteinizing hormone secreted by the anterior pituitary gland.

ovum (*pl* **ova**) the mature, unfertilized female reproductive cell, which is roughly spherical with an outer membrane and a single nucleus.

paraphimosis constriction of the penis because of retraction of an abnormally tight foreskin, which contracts on the penis behind the glans and cannot be easily moved. Swelling and pain may be caused and usually circumcision is necessary to prevent a recurrence.

pelvic inflammatory disease (PID) an acute or chronic infection of the uterus, ovaries or Fallopian tubes. It is the result of infection elsewhere, e.g. in the appendix, which spreads, or one that is carried by the blood. It produces severe abdominal pain, which usually responds to antibiotics but surgery may sometimes be necessary to remove diseased tissue.

penis the male organ through which the urethra passes, carrying urine or semen. It is made up of tissue that is filled with blood during sexual arousal, producing an erection that enables penetration of the vagina and ejaculation of semen. The glans is the end part, normally covered by the foreskin (prepuce).

pessary 1. an instrument that fits into the vagina to treat a prolapse. **2.** a soft solid substance that is shaped for insertion into the vagina and contains drugs for some gynaecological disorder (also used for inducing labour).

phallus 1. the penis or a penis-like object. **2.** the term used for the embryonic penis before the final development of the urethra.

phimosis a condition in which the edge of the foreskin is narrowed and cannot be drawn back over the glans of the penis. To avoid inflammation and an exacerbation of the problem, circumcision may be necessary.

placenta the organ attaching the embryo to the uterus. It is a temporary feature, comprising maternal and embryonic tissues, and it allows oxygen and nutrients to pass from the mother's blood to that of the embryo. There is, however, no direct contact of blood supplies. The embryo also receives salt, glucose, amino acids, some peptides and antibodies, fats and vitamins. Waste molecules from the embryo are removed by diffusion into the maternal circulation. It also stores glycogen for conversion to glucose, if required, and secretes hormones to regulate the pregnancy. It is expelled after birth.

placenta praevia the condition when the placenta is situated in the bottom part of the uterus next to or over the cervix. In the later stages of pregnancy there may be placental separation, causing bleeding that will require attention. In the more extreme cases, a Caesarean section is necessary for delivery.

postpartum the term meaning 'relating to the first few days after birth'.

pre-eclampsia the development of high blood pressure in pregnancy, sometimes with oedema, which, unless treated, may result in eclampsia.

pregnancy the period of time, lasting approximately 280 days from the first day of the last menstrual period, during which a woman carries a developing foetus. Signs of a pregnancy include cessation of menstruation, increase in size of the breasts, morning sickness and, later, the obvious sign of enlargement of the abdomen. A foetal heartbeat and movements can also be detected. Many of these changes are hormone-controlled, by progesterone (from the ovary and placenta).

pregnancy test any of various tests used to check for pregnancy, most of which are based on the presence of chorionic gonadotrophic hormone in the urine.

premature birth a birth occurring before the end of the normal full term of pregnancy. The definition refers to babies weighing less than 2.5 kg. In many cases the cause is unknown, but in some it may be because of pre-eclampsia, kidney or heart disease or multiple pregnancy. Premature babies often require incubator care.

premenstrual tension (PMT) *or* **premenstrual syndrome (PMS)** the occurrence for up to ten days before menstruation of such symptoms as headache, nervousness and irritability, emotional disturbance, depression, fatigue with other physical manifestations such as swelling of legs and breasts, and constipation. The condition usually disappears soon after menstruation begins. The cause is not known, although the hormone progesterone is probably involved in some way.

presentation the point, during labour, at which some part of the foetus lies at the mouth of the uterus.

progesterone a steroid hormone that is vital in pregnancy. It is produced by the corpus luteum of the ovary when the lining of the uterus is prepared for the implanting of an egg cell. Progesterone is secreted under the control of other hormones (prolactin from the anterior pituitary gland and luteinizing hormone also from the pituitary, which stimulates ovulation and formation of the corpus luteum) until the placenta adopts this role later in the pregnancy. The function of progesterone is to maintain the uterus and ensure that no further eggs are produced. Small amounts of this hormone are also produced by the testes.

prostaglandin (**PG**) any of a group of compounds, derived from essential fatty acids, that act in a way that is similar to hormones. They are found in most body tissues (but especially semen), where they are released as local regulators (in the uterus, brain, lungs, etc). A number have been identified, two of which act antagonistically on blood vessels, PGE causing dilation, PGF constriction. Certain prostaglandins cause contraction of the uterus in labour, and others are involved in the body's defence mechanisms.

prostatectomy surgical excision of the prostate gland, performed to relieve urine retention caused by enlargement of the prostate. It is also done to counter poor flow of urine or frequent urination. The operation can be undertaken from several approaches: via the urethra, from the bladder, or from the perineum (for a biopsy).

prostate gland a gland in the male reproductive system that is located below the bladder, opening into the urethra. Upon ejaculation, it secretes an alkaline fluid into the semen, which aids sperm motility. In older men, the gland may become enlarged, causing problems with urination.

prostatitis inflammation of the prostate gland as a result of bacterial infection. The symptoms tend to be similar to a urinary infection although in the chronic form obstructions may form, necessitating prostatectomy.

pubic pertaining to the pubes e.g. pubic hair.

pubis (*pl* **pubes**) one of the three bones, and the most anterior, that make up each half of the pelvic girdle.

puerperal fever an infection, now rare in developed countries, that occurs within two or three days of childbirth when a mother is susceptible to disease. Preventive measures are vital, but infections respond to antibiotic treatment.

quickening the first movements of a baby in the womb (uterus), which are perceived by the mother usually around the fourth month of pregnancy.

recessive gene a gene the character of which will only be expressed if paired with a similar gene (allele).

reproductive system the name given to all the organs involved in reproduction. In males these comprise the testicles, vasa deferentia, prostate gland, seminal vesicles, urethra and penis. In females, the reproductive system consists of the ovaries, Fallopian tubes, uterus, vagina and vulva.

safe period the days in a woman's menstrual cycle when conception is least likely. Ovulation usually occurs midway through the cycle, about 15 days before onset of menstruation, and the fertile period is about 5 days before and 5 after ovulation. Providing periods are regular, it can be calculated when intercourse is unlikely to result in pregnancy but it is an unreliable method of contraception.

scrotum the sac that contains the testicles and holds them outside the body to permit production and storage of sperm at a temperature lower than that of the abdomen.

secondary sexual characteristics the physical features that develop at puberty. In girls, the breasts and genitals increase in size and pubic hair grows. Boys grow pubic hair and facial hair, the voice breaks and the genitals become adult size.

semen the fluid that contains the sperm, which is ejaculated from the penis during sexual intercourse.

sex-linked disorders conditions produced because the genes controlling certain characteristics are carried on the sex chromosomes, usually the X-chromosome. Some result from an abnormal number of chromosomes, e.g. Klinefelter's syndrome affecting only men, and Turner's syndrome affecting only women. Other disorders, such as haemophilia, are carried on the X-chromosome and these manifest themselves in men because, although the genes are recessive, there is no other X-chromosome to mask the recessive type, as is the case with women.

sexually transmitted diseases (STDs) *or* **venereal diseases** diseases transmitted by sexual intercourse. These include HIV/AIDS, syphilis, gonorrhoea, nonspecific urethritis, etc.

sperm the mature male reproductive cell or gamete. It has a head with the haploid nucleus containing half the chromosome number and an acrosome (a structure that aids penetration of the egg). Behind the head comes a midpiece with energy-producing mitochondria, and then a long tail that propels it forward. A few millilitres of semen is ejaculated during sexual intercourse, containing many millions of sperm.

spermatic the term given to any vessel or structure associated with the testicle.

spermatozoon (*pl* **spermatozoa**) the scientific name for sperm.

spermicide a cream, foam, jelly, etc, that kills sperm and is used in conjunction with a diaphragm as a contraceptive.

sterilization a surgical operation to render someone incapable of producing children. Men usually undergo a vasectomy while in women it can be achieved by cutting and tying the Fallopian tubes or removing them. The latter operation is performed via an incision in the abdominal wall or through the vagina.

stillbirth the birth of any child that provides no evidence of life.

syphilis an infectious, sexually transmitted disease caused by the bacterium Treponema pallidum. Treatment of syphilis is with penicillin early in the development of the disease.

testicle *or* **testis** (*pl* **testes**) one of the pair of male sex organs that are situated within the scrotum and produce sperm and secrete the hormone testosterone. The testicles develop within the abdomen of the foetus but descend around the time of birth into the scrotum. Each testicle has an outer double membrane layer, known as the tunica vaginalis. The tunica vaginalis contains an inner fibrous layer, called the tunica albuginea, which protects the testicle. The bulk of the testicle consists of numerous fine, convoluted tubules called seminiferous tubules, which are lined with cells that produce the sperm. In addition, other cells, known as sertoli cells, occur, which provide support and possibly nourishment for the developing sperm. The tubules are supported by connective tissue containing nerves and blood vessels and also the cells of Leydig, which are responsible for hormone production. The tubules connect with another highly folded tube, called the epididymis, which is about 7m long and connects with the vas deferens, which leads to the urethra. The spermatozoa are passed by passive movement along the epididymis, completing their development as they go, and are stored in the lower part until ejaculation.

testosterone the male sex hormone secreted by the testes.

thrush an infection caused by the fungus Candida albicans, which affects the mucous membranes of the mouth and vagina, producing white patches. It is a popular name given to a group of infections known as candidiasis.

urethra the duct carrying urine from the bladder out of the body. It is about 3.5 cm long in women and 20 cm in men. The male urethra runs through the penis and also forms the ejaculatory duct.

urethritis inflammation of the mucous lining of the urethra, which may be associated with cystitis, often being the cause of the latter. The commonest cause of urethritis is gonorrhoea (specific urethritis). Alternatively, it may be caused by infection with microorganisms (nonspecific urethritis). Sulphonamide and antibiotic drugs are effective once the infecting organism is identified.

urinogenital a collective term describing all organs and tissues involved in excretion and reproduction because they are closely linked anatomically and functionally.

uterus *or* **womb** a roughly pear-shaped organ within the cavity of the pelvis that is specialized for the growth and nourishment of a foetus. Fallopian tubes connect to the upper part and the lower part joins the vagina at the cervix. It has a plentiful blood supply along with lymphatic vessels and nerves. During pregnancy it enlarges considerably and the smooth muscle walls thicken. Contractions of the muscular wall push the foetus out via the vagina at childbirth. If there is no pregnancy, the lining undergoes periodic changes (menstruation).

vagina the lower part of the female reproductive tract that leads from the uterus to the outside. It receives the erect penis during sexual intercourse, the semen being ejaculated into the upper part from where the sperm pass through the cervix and uterus to the Fallopian tubes. The vagina is essentially a muscular tube lined with mucous membrane.

vaginitis inflammation of the vagina as a result of infection or deficiency in diet or poor hygiene. There may be itching, a discharge and pain on urination.

vas deferens (*pl* **vasa deferentia**) one of the two tubes that join the testes to the ejaculatory duct via the prostate gland.

vasectomy the cutting of the vas deferens, which is performed on both ducts, causing sterility, although the effect is not immediate.

vulva (*pl* **vulvae**) the external female genitalia, comprising two pairs of fleshy folds (labia) surrounding the opening of the vagina. Below them is the clitoris.

vulvectomy surgical removal of the vulva. The extent of the operation depends on whether there is a malignant or non-malignant growth.

vulvitis inflammation of the vulva.

vulvovaginitis inflammation of both the vulva and vagina.

X-chromosome the sex chromosome present in males and females, although women have a pair and men just one (with one Y-chromosome). Certain disorders, such as haemophilia, are carried as genes on the X-chromosome.

Y-chromosome the small sex chromosome that carries a dominant gene conferring maleness. Normal males have 22 matched chromosome pairs and one unmatched pair, comprising one X-chromosome and one Y-chromosome. During sexual reproduction, the mother contributes an X-chromosome, but the father contributes an X or Y-chromosome. XX produces a female offspring and XY a male.